2

Edoardo Foce
Endo-periodontal Lesions

Edoardo Foce

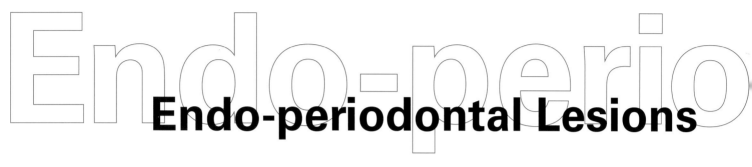

Endo-periodontal Lesions

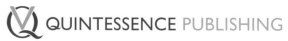 QUINTESSENCE PUBLISHING

London, Berlin, Chicago, Tokyo, Barcelona, Beijing, Istanbul, Milan, Moscow, New Delhi, Paris, Prague, São Paulo, Seoul and Warsaw

First published in Italian in 2009 by Quintessenza Edizioni, Milan:
Lesioni Endo-parodontali.

Quintessence
British Library Cataloguing in Publication Data
Foce, Edoardo.
Endo-periodontal lesions.
1. Periodontics. 2. Endodontics. 3. Periodontal disease
Diagnosis. 4. Periodontal disease Treatment. 5. Dental pulp
Diseases Diagnosis. 6. Dental pulp Diseases Treatment.
I. Title
617.6'3-dc22
ISBN-13: 9781850972105

Quintessence Publishing Co. Ltd,
Grafton Road, New Malden, Surrey KT3 3AB,
Great Britain
www.quintpub.co.uk
Copyright © 2011 by Quintessence Publishing Co. Ltd

Editing: Quintessence Publishing Co. Ltd, Chicago
Layout and Production: Quintessenz Verlags-GmbH, Berlin, Germany
Printed and bound in Germany by Bosch Druck GmbH

Dedications

To my wife, Lilly and son, Alessandro — this book may have robbed you of some of my time but not one ounce of my love;

to my sister Giovanna, with whom I silently treasure both memories and the present;

to my mother Milla, with immense love, respect, and gratitude;

and especially to my father, Dr Gianfranco, to whom I would have wished to present my first book with pride and thankfulness, but who is no longer with us and whose loss is with me constantly.

Acknowledgments

My sincere gratitude goes to all those from whom I have learned, in particular Dr Arnaldo Castellucci, Dr Fabio Gorni, and Dr Gianfranco Carnevale, without whose guidance this work probably would never have happened.

I am grateful to my colleagues and friends, Dr Augusto Malentacca, Dr Mario Badino, Dr Piero Alessandro Marcoli, and Prof Elio Berutti for kindly permitting me to use their documentation.

Special thanks are due to Grazia Innocenti for her extraordinary professional skill, patience, and acumen in arranging and enhancing the layout, text, and images.

My keen appreciation goes to my office administrator, Lorenza Garosi and my hygienist, Dr Roberta Russo.

Sincere thanks go to all my patients.

I am indebted to Dr Piero Biaggini and his firm for all of their moral and logistic support and assistance.

Finally, I owe much to Gianfranco Cavallo, who spurred me on tirelessly to develop on this theme.

Foreword

The subject of combined endo-perio lesions is surrounded by considerable confusion. One frequently hears diagnoses of endo-perio lesions when in fact there is an endodontic lesion mimicking periodontal disease or, vice versa, a purely periodontal lesion perfectly is camouflaged as an endodontic pathology. This occurs as a result of the similarity of their signs and symptoms, given that both diseases and their resulting lesions affect the same area, namely the tooth-support apparatus that is comprised of the cementum, periodontal ligament, and bone.

Therefore, I have great pleasure in recommending this work by Dr Edoardo Foce not only to undergraduates and graduates but, above all, to clinicians who practice our profession. This book offers a significant advantage in that Dr Foce has finally thrown light on a subject that until now was often confused or misinterpreted. His new classification system, accompanied by abundant clinical case documentation, provides a starting point for correct diagnosis and consequently a successful treatment plan.

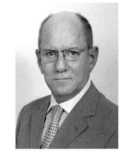

My sincere congratulations go to my friend and colleague, Dr Foce for having produced a text illustrating with rare clarity on such a complex and often-debated subject while also highlighting the importance of interdisciplinary knowledge. Periodontology goes hand-in-hand with endodontics, conservative dentistry, prosthodontics, implant dentistry, and oral surgery.

Dr Arnaldo Castellucci

Foreword

This work by Dr Edoardo Foce stands apart from other single-author books or chapters on this subject thanks to the clinical approach he has chosen.

I find the new classification proposed by the author highly interesting and logical, especially in the light of its impact on how to proceed with treatment. It is my opinion that the endo-perio area has until now been complicated by hazy classifications often having little in common with reality.

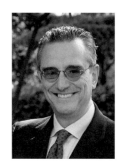

Dr Foce's decision to present emblematic cases illustrating the correlations between endodontium and periodontium appears intelligent and eminently practical since the book provides many ideas and suggestions concerning the connections not only between endodontics and periodontics but also between endodontics and all the other dental specialties involving the periodontium, including conservative dentistry, oral surgery, and prosthodontics.

Dr Gianfranco Carnevale

Table of Contents

Introduction

The human periodontium and dental pulp cavity are closely connected by their proximity and by the presence of apical and lateral radicular foramina, which permit the passage of pathogens between these two distinct anatomical areas (Fig 1). The pulp-periodontal interrelationship is one in which "there are so many paths of communication that one is tempted to put aside the notion of two distinct anatomical structures and consider them as a single continuous system."[1]

Nomenclature distinguishes between lesions caused by periodontal pathogens, as seen in chronic periodontitis, and disorders of the apical periodontal tissues associated with endodontic pathology. When the location is distinct and the lesion is discrete, the two are easy to differentiate (Fig 2).

Other pathologic profiles exist that, as shown by clinical and radiologic examination, simultaneously affect the marginal and apical areas of the periodontium, thus making it essential to ascertain their true cause through differential diagnosis (Fig 3). The expression *endo-perio lesion*[2] was devised to better describe the etiopathogenesis in such cases and includes lesions:

• Caused by endodontic pathogens that have spread coronally, thus involving the gingival margin and in some cases creating a fistula, or *sinus tract*
• Originating from a marginal lesion which has subsequently affected more apical periodontal areas

• Resulting from of a combination of the above, in which case the differential diagnosis must attribute each portion of the lesion to its cause (Fig 4)

Because chronic endo-perio lesions are common in clinical practice, a number of authors have already addressed this issue.[1,3–9] This contribution has been added because the term *endo-perio lesion* can often be unclear and merits further elaboration. When one fails to distinguish clearly among varying pathologies, one falls into the trap of lumping them together, defeating the purpose of much research and literature.

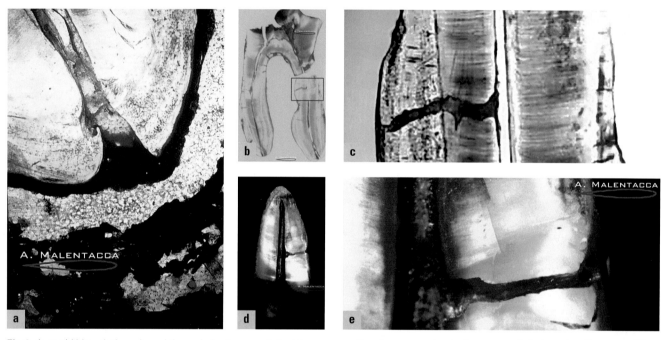

Fig 1 *(a to e)* Although the pulp and the periodontium are distinct from one another, they are anatomically connected via foramina. (Courtesy of Dr Augusto Malentacca.)

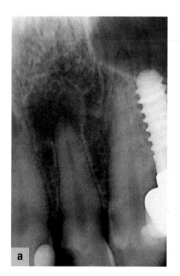

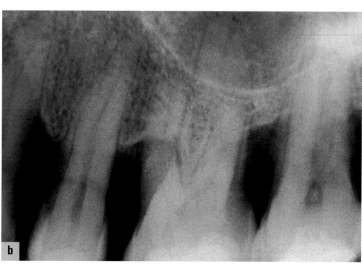

Fig 2 *(a)* An apical lesion of endodontic origin. *(b)* Attachment and bone loss in the alveolar crest area.

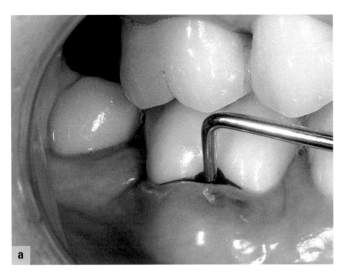
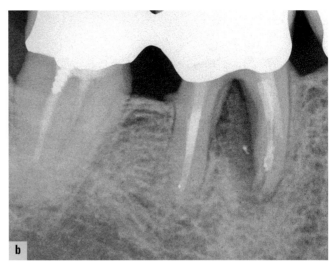

Fig 3 *(a and b)* Clinical and radiologic investigation of the marginal and more apical periodontium, highlighting the need for a differential diagnostic approach to uncover the true nature of the lesion's endo-perio status.

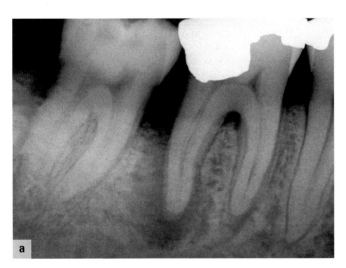

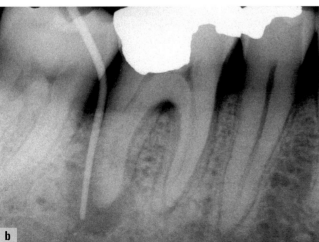
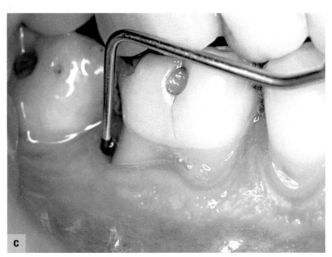

Fig 4 *(a to c)* Clinical and radiologic examinations show marginal and apical periodontal involvement, making it necessary to ascertain the true nature of the lesion.

Chapter One
Terminology

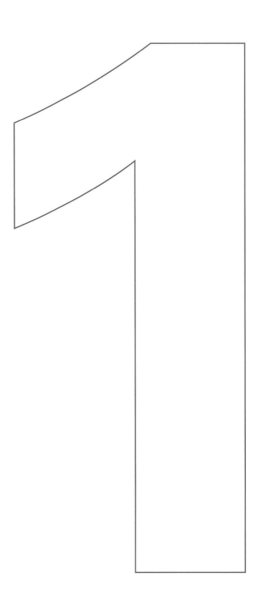

Terminology, by nature, implies a consensus in regards to the terms used to define a given thing, person, or concept. This brings to mind the famous quote from Umberto Eco's *The Name of the Rose*: "Stat rosa pristina nomine, nomina nuda tenemus (what is left of the rose is only its name)."[10]

In the English language the first word in expressions such as *bone injuries*, *cardiac lesions*, or *brain damage* clearly denotes which part of the body is affected. As a logical extension of this concept, the expression *endo-perio lesions* should be interpreted as meaning that the lesions in question are present in both the pulp cavity and the periodontium. While this is in itself correct and precisely describes the affected parts, it is problematic that the term is often misinterpreted as a reference to the etiopathogenesis, or origin. This misunderstanding is usually implied rather than directly stated.

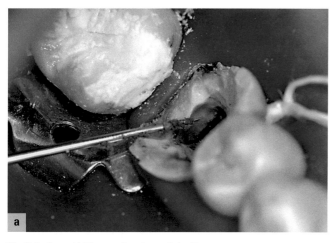
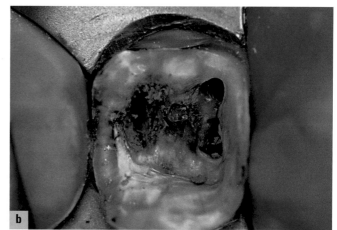

Fig 1-1 *(a and b)* Decayed root canal dentin.

Fig 1-2 *(a and b)* Pulp with capillary congestion shown by copious bleeding once the chamber was opened.

Fig 1-3 *(a and b)* Pus exudating along with necrotized canal tissue.

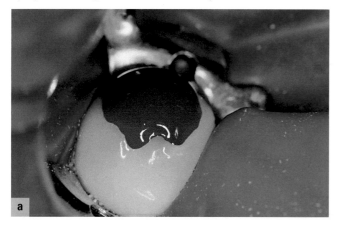
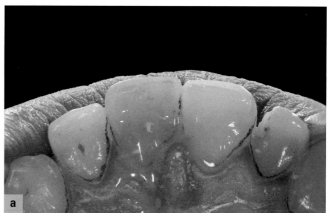

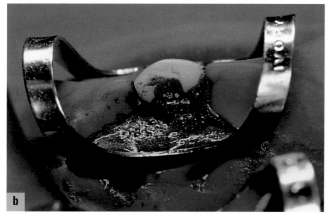
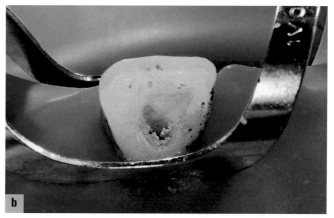

Endodontic Lesions

If the words of the expression *endo-perio lesions* are rearranged, the resulting phrase *endodontic lesions* unintentionally omits a reference to a potential origin of the pathology that is vital for correct diagnosis and treatment: in this case the periodontium. To discuss endodontic lesions without clarifying the source of the disorder or to take knowledge of that source for granted can create a misunderstanding because the phrase *endodontic lesion* automatically refers to pathologies of the pulp.

The term *endodontic* is also understood as implying etiology and is often used in connection with endodontic pathologies that gives rise to a lesion affecting a different structure, namely the periodontium.

There are many examples of this class of pathologic changes:

- Decay within the root canal (Fig 1-1)
- Hyperemia (Fig 1-2) and pulp necrosis (Fig 1-3)
- Calcification (Fig 1-4)
- Sclerosis (Fig 1-5)
- Internal resorption (Figs 1-6 and 1-7)

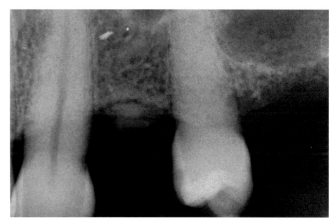

Fig 1-5 Sclerosis has radiologically obliterated the canal.

Fig 1-6 *(a and b)* The mandibular left first molar shows areas of internal resorption in the mesial and distal roots. Note how the endodontic filler has satisfactorily filled the areas of resorption.

Fig 1-4 *(a and b)* Large stone in the pulp chamber.

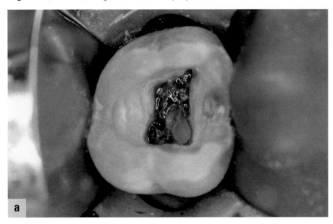

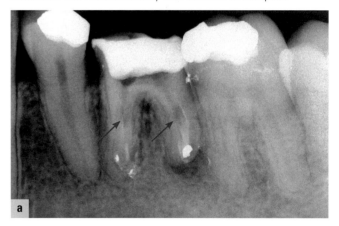

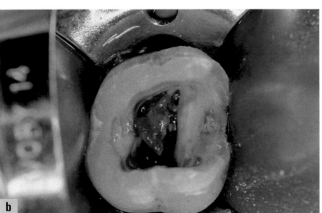

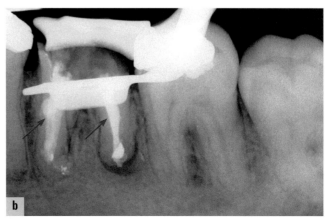

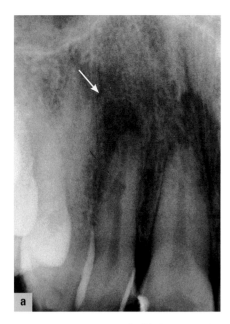

Fig 1-7 Maxillary right lateral incisor with pulp necrosis, apical lesion, and internal resorption affecting the middle third of the root. The chronic apical inflammation, shown by the corresponding area of radiolucency, has caused resorption at the apical foramen, leading to leakage of filler despite use of a large gutta-percha cone. *(a)* The internal resorption *(red arrow)* is an endodontic lesion in that it originates from and is situated in the pulp. The periodontal lesion *(white arrow)* is an apical granuloma that is situated in and develops in periodontal tissue. The term *periodontal lesion* here refers precisely to its location, not its cause. *(b)* Note the position of the instrument *(red arrow)* placed at the apex of the canal (working length) that, in this case, terminates apically higher than the root apex. *(c)* The gutta-percha cone *(white arrow)* is intentionally placed approximately 1 mm shorter than the working length at the end of the canal. *(d)* The entire canal system is sealed with thermoplasticized gutta percha *(red arrow),* and the tooth crown is reconstructed with composite. *(e to g)* Follow-up posttreatment radiographs taken at 4, 6, and 8 years, respectively, indicate that the internal resorption area appears stable. Despite imperfect control of the sealant at the apex, there are no visible signs of lesions.

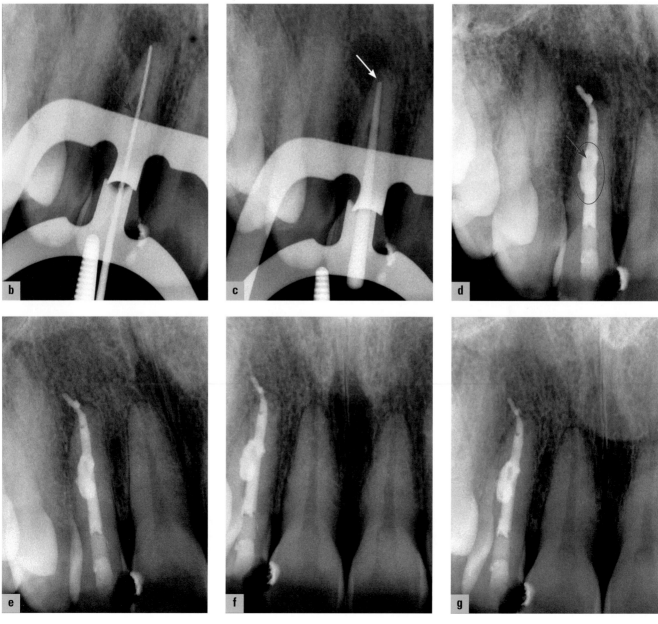

Periodontal Lesions

In the expression *periodontal lesions*, the term *periodontal* also has two concurrent meanings. The first, literal meaning indicates the position of the lesion, while the second refers to its etiopathogenesis, be it periodontal or endodontic tissues. This lack of terminological clarity may cause confusion.

Firstly, one must be aware of the variety and multi-faceted nature of the pathogenic factors capable of producing lesions in the periodontium, as well as the differences between these same lesions in anatomical-pathologic terms. The most common causes of periodontal disease are, of course, dental plaque and calculus. Conditions able to provoke periodontal lesions in a previously healthy periodontium include occlusal trauma, vertical root fracture, and caries spreading along the external root surface under the cementoenamel junction (CEJ). In addition to traumatic or pathogenic factors, periodontal lesions may also be caused iatrogenically: orthodontic tooth movement, scaling and root planing and other dental hygiene procedures, perio-

dontal surgery, subgingival implants, and gingival retraction cords.

When the term *periodontal* is used to describe a pathogenic factor rather than an anatomical location, it is often associated with those lesions that, from a histopathologic point of view, are typified by a loss of connective attachment and consequent apical migration of the junctional epithelium.

While these symptoms are characteristic of lesions occurring in the periodontium as a result of periodontal disorders, they may also be associated directly or indirectly with other conditions including:

- Vertical root fractures (Figs 1-8 and 1-9)
- Root abnormalities such as:
  - Irregularly developed grooves (Fig 1-10)
  - Enamel pearls in various positions (Fig 1-11)[11,12]
- Internal perforating root resorption (with the lesion extending to the surface)
- Extracanal invasive resorption (Fig 1-12)[13]
- External cervical root resorption (Fig 1-13)[14,15]

Fig 1-8 *(a to d)* Maxillary right second premolar with vertical root fracture. On initial investigation, probing may indicate exactly the same signs as those of a sinus tract caused by intraligament drainage of an endodontic lesion. For this reason, it is essential to ascertain the exact cause, in this case a fracture, with accuracy.

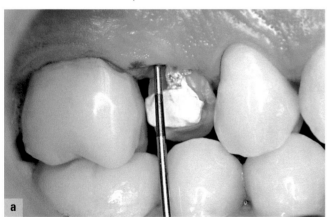

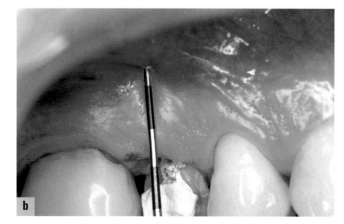

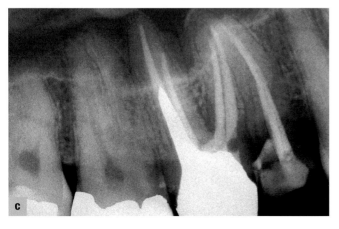

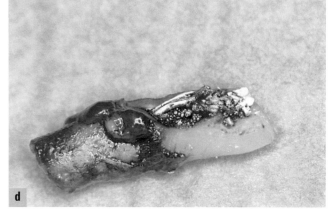

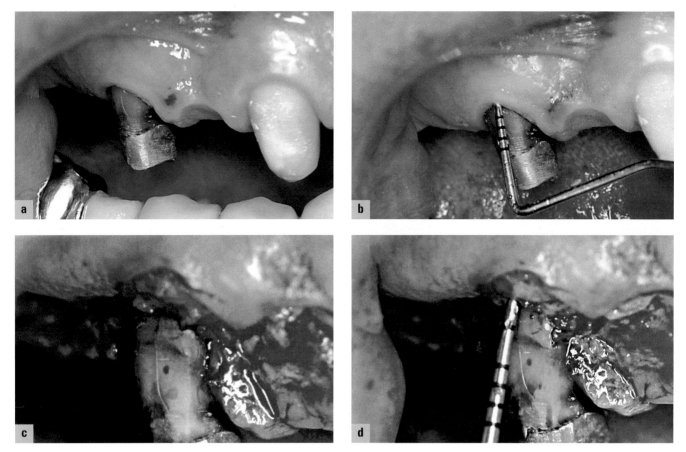

Fig 1-9 *(a to d)* Under certain conditions, detection of a fracture with a probe may present additional difficulties if structures interfere with the proper route of the probe.

Fig 1-10 Maxillary left lateral incisor with a distolingual groove of moderate depth. *(a)* Preoperative radiograph. *(b)* Groove visible distal to the cingulum. *(c)* Probing of the defect reaches approx 5 mm. *(d)* Postoperative radiograph. (Courtesy of Dr Arnaldo Castellucci.)

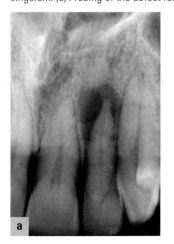
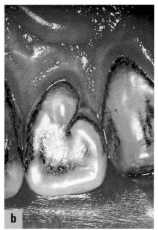
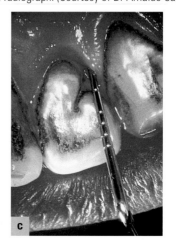
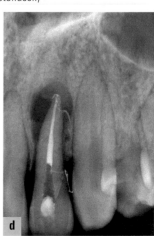

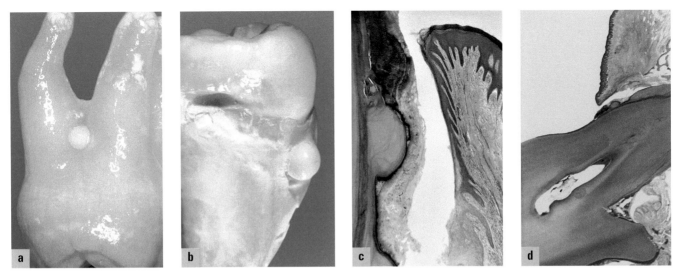

Fig 1-11 Enamel pearls. *(a)* Enamel pearl in the buccal furcation of a maxillary first molar. *(b)* Enamel pearl on the buccal surface of a mandibular molar. *(c)* Enamel pearl on the distal surface of the distal root of a third molar. *(d)* Magnification of a periodontal defect corresponding to the pearl. (Courtesy of Prof A. Bloom.)

Figs 1-12a to 1-12e Extracanal invasive resorption affecting the mesial side of the palatal root of a maxillary right first molar.[13]

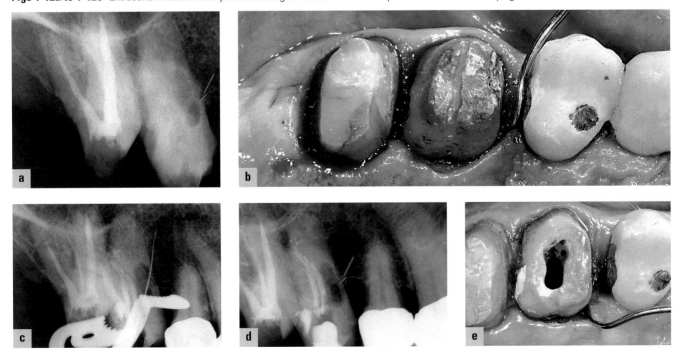

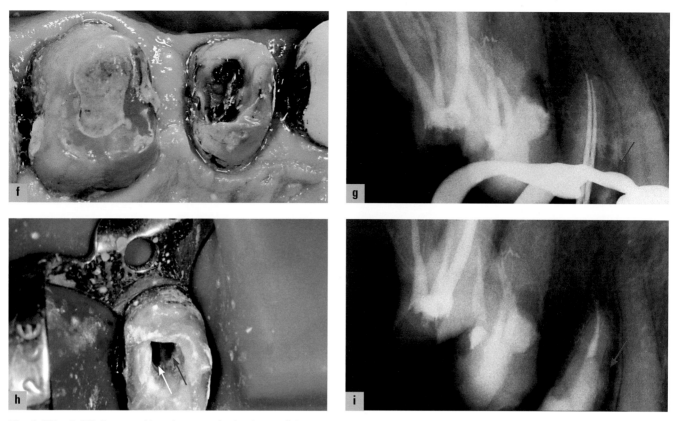

Figs 1-12f to 1-12i Extracanal invasive resorption (*red arrows*) also present on the mesial surface in the area of the interradicular concavity of a neighboring maxillary right first premolar. The white arrow is showing the root canal.

Figs 1-12j to 1-12n *(j to l)* During osseous resective surgery, an osseous defect correlating to root resorption is discovered mesial to the maxillary first premolar. *(m and n)* The extent of resorption is visible on the extracted tooth. This is another context that would justify the use of the term *endo-perio* to define the disorder.

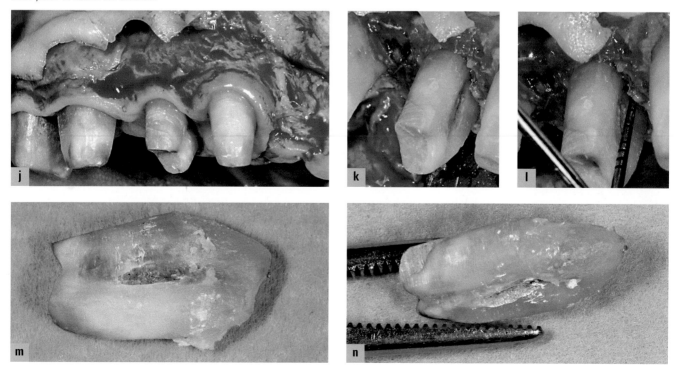

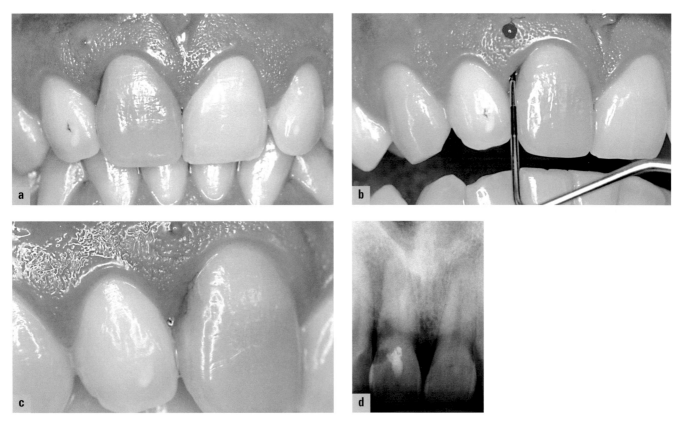

Figs 1-13a to 1-13d Class 3 cervical resorption.[15,16]

Figs 1-13e to 1-13j Because the lesion had spread and caused pulpitis, endodontic treatment was completed.

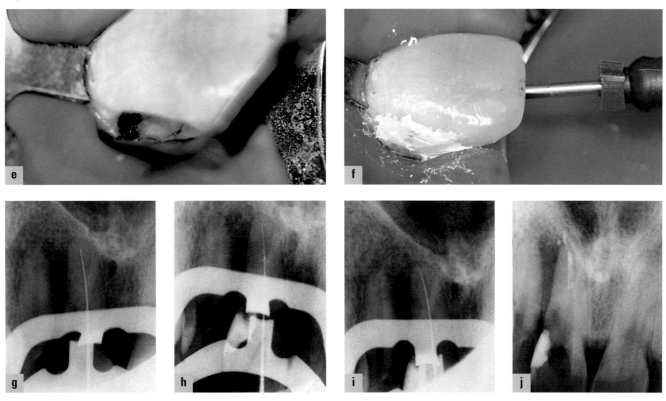

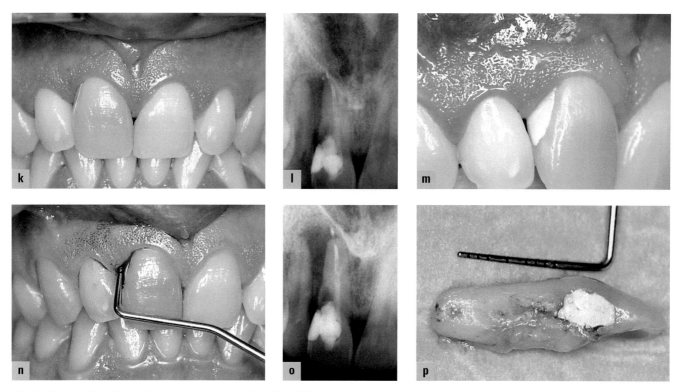

Figs 1-13k to 1-13p *(k to m)* Despite being warned, the patient failed to present for follow-up once the endodontic treatment had eliminated painful symptoms. *(n to p)* When the pain returned a year later, radiographic examination showed Class 4 invasive marginal resorption.

Figs 1-13q to 1-13v This severe plaque-induced periodontal lesion with associated destruction of root tissue indicated extraction of the tooth. Despite grafting of osteoconductive material into the postoperative site, the healing stage was marked by significant labial bone resorption.[17]

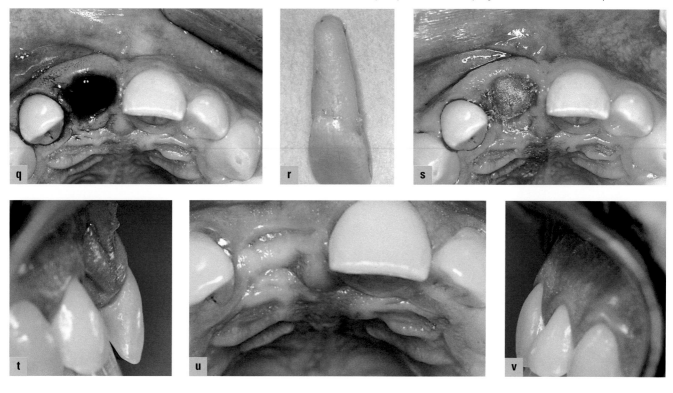

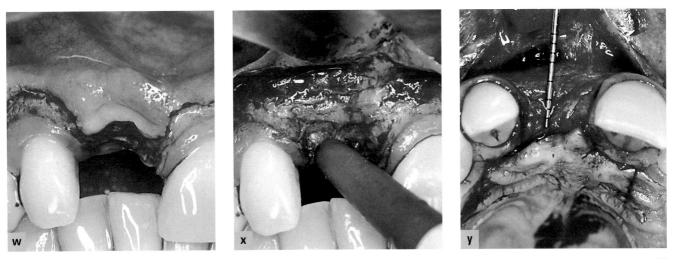

Figs 1-13w to 1-13y Morphologic and functional rehabilitation of the edentulous site indicated placement of an implant following ridge expansion.[18]

Figs 1-13z to 1-13ee Stages of surgical correction and implant placement include use of a scalpel with beaver blade, a CV series bone expander, and an Exacta implant (Biaggini).

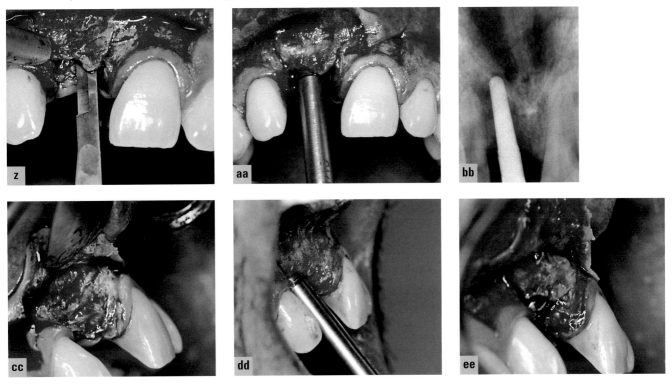

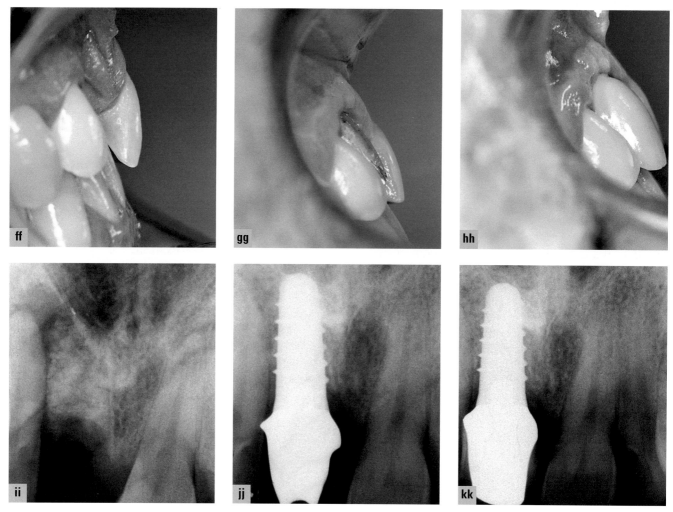

Figs 1-13ff to 1-13kk Following the ridge expansion there is a visible improvement in labial osseous contours in the area of the implant.

Figs 1-13ll to 1-13oo Pretreatment and posttreatment conditions.

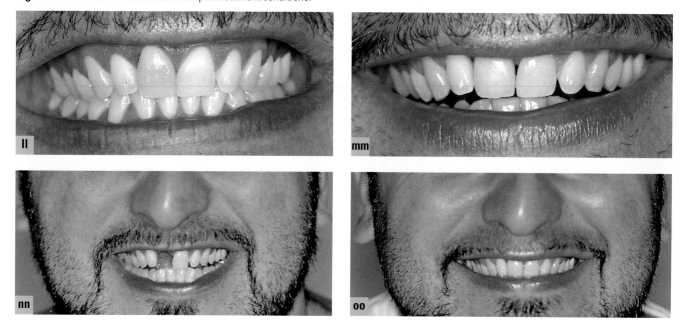

From both a diagnostic and operational perspective it is essential to consider endo-perio relations (see Figs 1-12j to 1-12n). Failure to take these into due consideration may, for example, result in proceeding with regenerating treatment on the grounds that an intrabony defect seemed a perfect surgical candidate in light of its location, width, depth, angle and number of remaining walls. Recognizing the endo-perio origin of a lesion should guide treatment decision making.

Lesions provoked in the periodontium, in addition to the various diseases and disorders listed on page 9, may also be associated with or caused by:

- Caries affecting the external root surface below the CEJ (Figs 1-14 and 1-15).[19–22]
- Iatrogenic causes such as restoration margins (Figs 1-16 and 1-17) and prosthetic devices (Fig 1-18), which may affect the external root surface apical to the CEJ and invade the biologic width. This damage may spread to apically located tissues.[19–22]

The interproximal areas in Fig 1-18 show the periodontal attachment apparatus following apically the scalloping of the CEJs. By their embryologic nature, the supracrestal fibers in a healthy undamaged periodontium insert into the radicular cementum situated just below the enamel. The physiologic architecture of the interproximal area means that the attachment level in the buccal and palatolingual areas is more apical than in the interproximal areas. This creates a convex coronal shape known as *physiologic* or *positive* architecture. Should this area be affected by caries or iatrogenic causes leading to loss of attachment apparatus and consequent apical migration of the CEJ, the positive architecture will be lost. The interproximal fibers will insert into the radicular cementum further apically than in the buccal and lingual attachment apparatus. The resulting shape is defined as *inverted* or *negative* architecture. From a practical point of view, this altered, concave shape is difficult to clean and favors the onset of soft tissue craters.

Fig 1-14 *(a to f)* Relationship between carious damage and periodontal margin attachment.

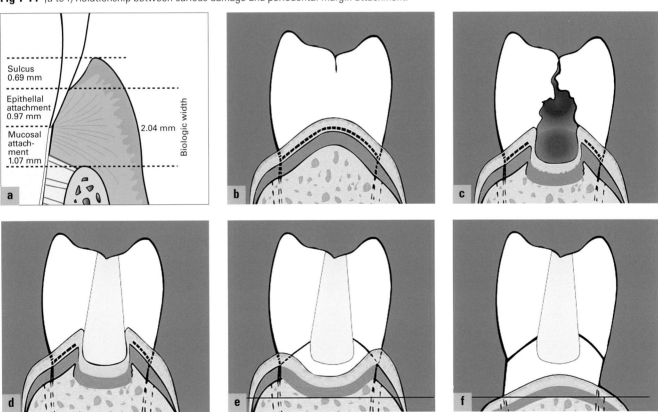

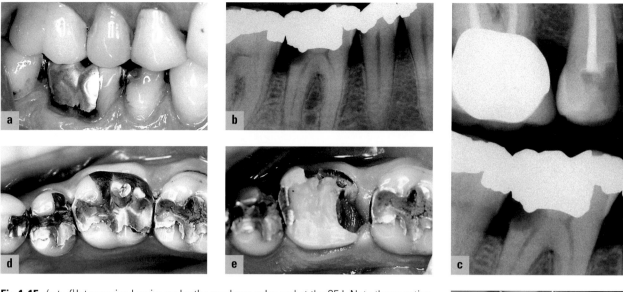

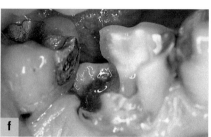

Fig 1-15 *(a to f)* Interproximal caries under the amalgam onlay and at the CEJ. Note the negative architecture and soft tissue crater. Since interdental gingival tissues are supported coronally by the buccal and lingual attachment apparatus, destruction and apical regression of the connective fibers withdraw this support, leading to corresponding tissue collapse and the formation of craters.

Fig 1-16 *(a to i)* Conservative restorations and caries below the CEJ.

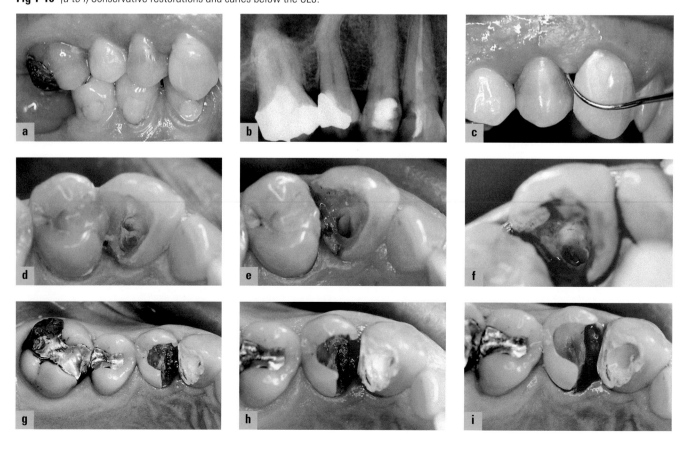

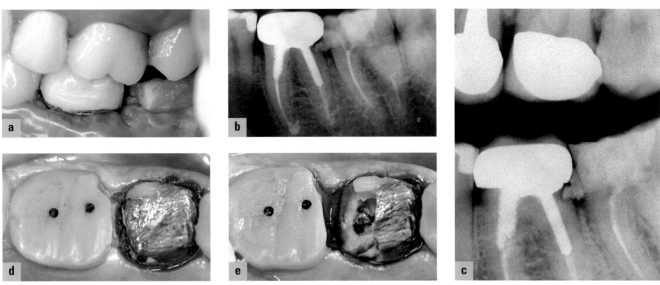

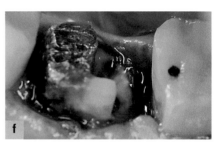

Fig 1-17 *(a to f)* A subgingival restoration has invaded the biologic width causing damage.

Fig 1-18 *(a to d)* Periodontal inflammation adjacent to the conservatively restored maxillary right second premolar and around the margin of the first premolar.

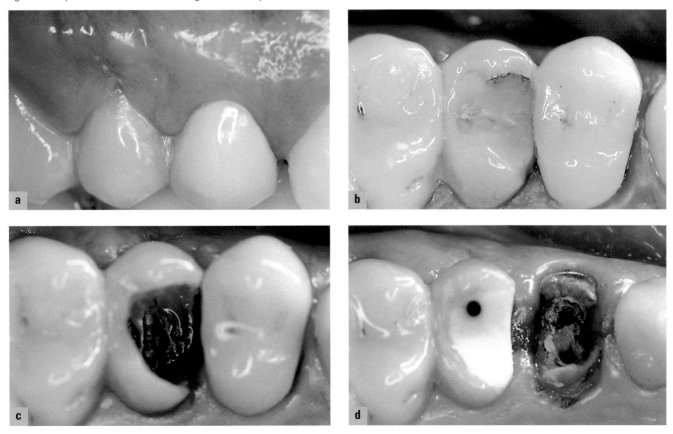

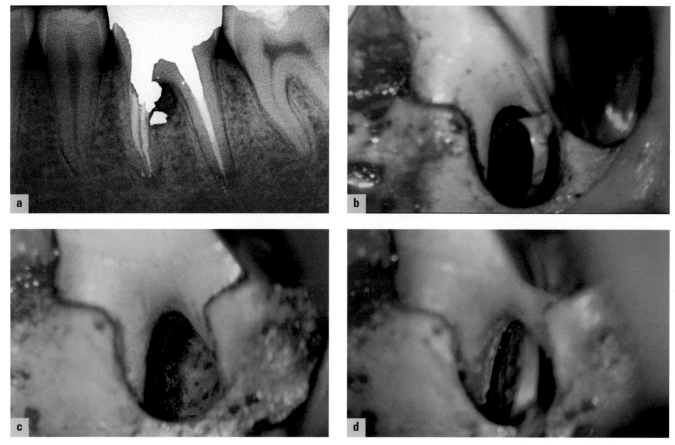

Figs 1-19a to 1-19d The mandibular left first molar presented with an endo-perio lesion caused by excessive stripping of the mesial canals into the furcation. *(a)* The radiograph highlights an attempt to repair the stripping damage with amalgam, and also shows an osseous defect at the furcation. Clinical examination revealed considerable probing depth along the entire buccal face, with maximum depth of 5 mm near the furcation. *(b)* In the surgical site, note the furcation defect and micromirror reflection of amalgam on the distal face of the mesial root. *(c)* Removal of amalgam and clearing of bone defect. *(d)* Stripping damage repaired with cement (Super Seal [Ogna]).

Figs 1-19e to 1-19g *(e and f)* Completed repair and placement of Gore-Tex membrane (WL Gore). *(g)* Postoperative control radiograph.

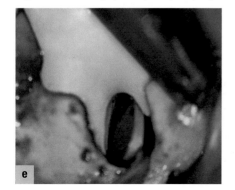
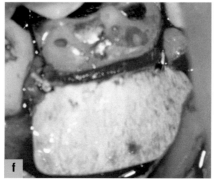
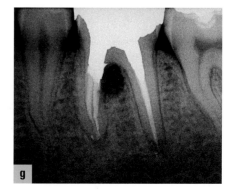

Summary

The importance of the correct use of terminology cannot be stressed enough. The expression *endo-perio* can be interpreted as referring to lesions in the periodontium as a result of either endodontic or periodontal pathology. Perforation and stripping (Figs 1-19 and 1-20) can cause periodontal lesions directly, but bear in mind that excessive or forceful use of instrumentation during root canal cleaning and shaping can frequently cause root fracture and consequently be an indirect cause of periodontal lesions.[23–26]

Any lesion produced in the periodontium by iatrogenic causes such as perforation, stripping, or forceful instrumentation is of endodontic origin. Application of a generalized interpretation of their etiopathogenesis would make it correct to define them as *endo-perio lesions*: periodontal lesions caused by endodontic treatment. Figures 1-20 and 1-21 illustrate practical examples.   ■

Figs 1-19h to 1-19j *(h)* Site reopened and membrane removed. Note abundance of newly formed tissue completely filling the furcal bone defect. *(i)* Soft tissues 6 months postoperation. *(j)* Ten-year follow-up radiograph. (Courtesy of Prof Elio Berutti.)

Figs 1-20a to 1-20c Instrument damage to distal root canal and presence of interradicular periodontal lesion.

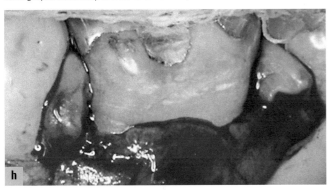

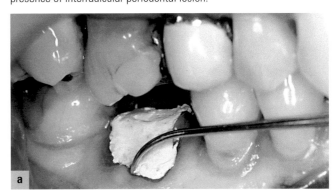

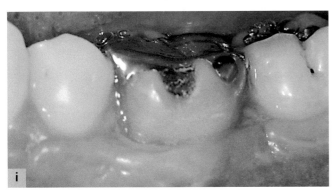

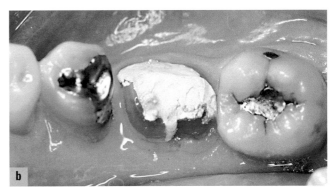

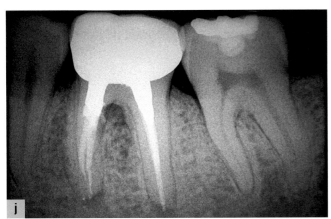

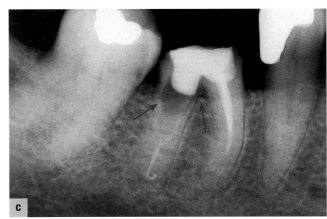

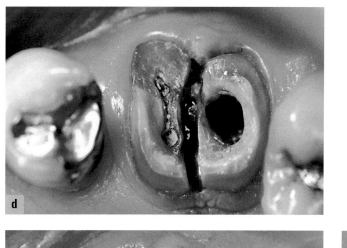

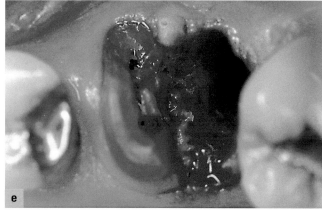

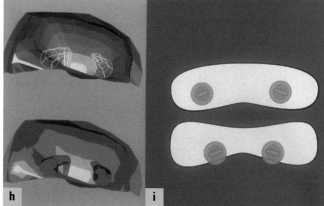

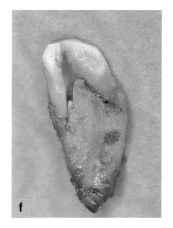
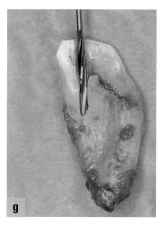

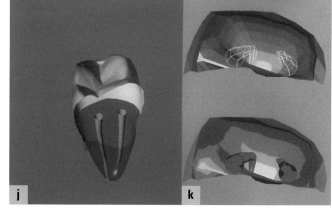

Figs 1-20d to 1-20g Iatrogenous perforation of the mandibular right first molar mesiolingual root concavity.

Figs 1-20h to 1-20k When using instruments to clean and shape root canals, as in this case, it is essential to predict the anatomical limits as well as the potential for damage of the procedures used.

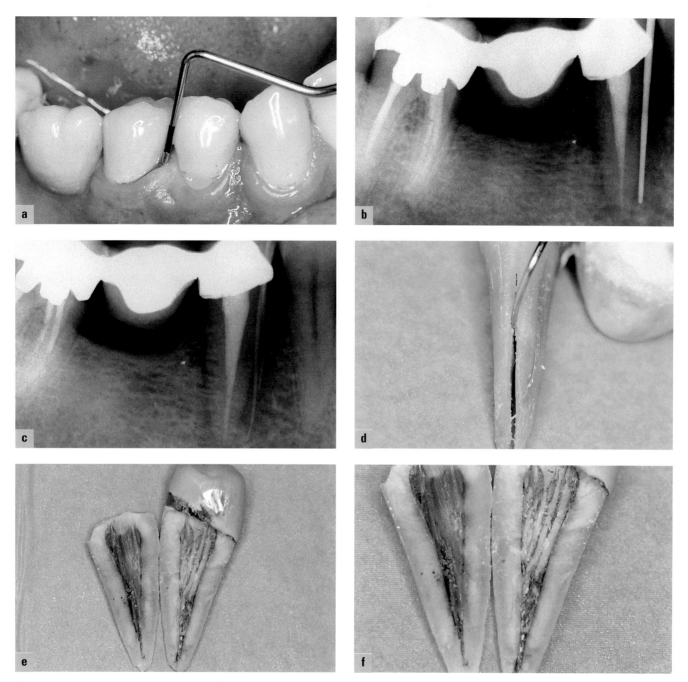

Fig 1-21 *(a to f)* Vertical fracture of the mandibular right second premolar, the abutment tooth for the patient's fixed partial denture. Excessive removal of root canal dentin, compounded by further removal of hard tissue when preparing the tooth as an abutment, probably contributed to coronal fracture.

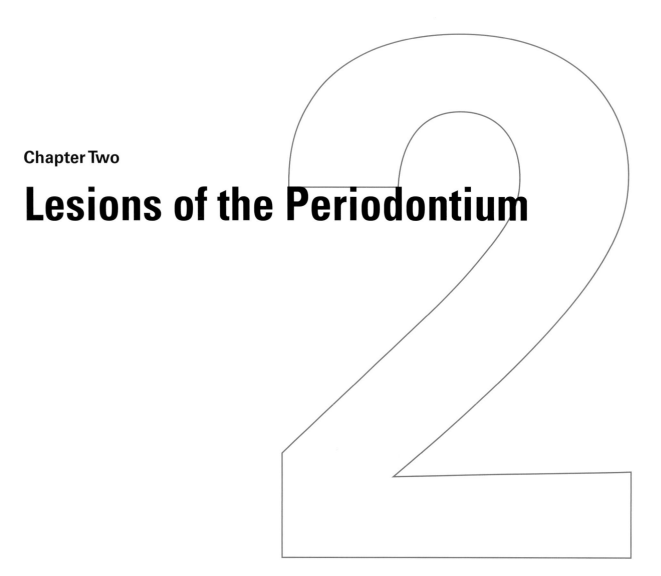

Chapter Two

Lesions of the Periodontium

Some periodontal lesions are endodontic in origin but have the histopathologic characteristics and infectious-inflammatory nature of *periodontitis* (inflammation of the teeth's supporting tissues).

Periodontal Lesions of Endodontic Origin

A periodontal lesion of endodontic origin arises when pathogens, toxins, and toxic metabolites present within the pulp cavity migrate through the apical and lateral periradicular foramina[27] and, according to some, through the dentinal tubules.[28–31] This provokes an inflammatory response as a defense against the invasion of the periodontium. Healthy periodontal tissue is replaced by inflammatory tissue. Radiologic and clinical examination will reveal a periodontal lesion of endodontic origin, typically at the root apex (Fig 2-1), but the lesion may extend along the lateral surface of the root (Fig 2-2) at points corresponding to the lateral canals and their respective foramina (Fig 2-3).

In multirooted teeth, these lesions may also develop in furcation areas (Figs 2-4 to 2-6) due to the presence of accessory canals linking the pulp cavity floor with the inter-radicular periodontium[5] (Fig 2-7). Lateral canals from the coronal and middle thirds of the radicular pulp cavity also extend to the furcation.[32–34] Some authors have observed that canals exiting the floor of the pulp cavity do not always have corresponding foramina in the furcation area.[35,36]

Pathology is more prevalent toward the apex. The apical foramen is the primary route of communication between periodontal tissues and the pulp. Furthermore, lateral canals and their foramina are more concentrated at the apex and, while present along the length of the root, decrease in number and size as the cementoenamel junction (CEJ) is approached (Figs 2-8 to 2-10).[37]

The periodontal response to endodontic pathology can range from mild inflammation to substantial destruction of the periodontium. Periodontal diagnoses can include chronic or acute apical periodontitis, acute apical abscess, draining sinus tract, and apical granuloma, among others. From an etiopathogenic standpoint, the development of these lesions may not be well correlated with the onset of endodontic infection.[6]

The *apical granuloma* is histologically characterized by the presence of inflammatory cell infiltrate, capillary buds, fibroblasts, and edema, usually surrounded by a capsule of connective tissue.[38,39] An apical granuloma results from *chronic apical periodontitis*, which is a result of persistent leakage of inflammatory-infective byproducts from a necrotic pulp. This nodule proliferates around the root apex and causes resorption of surrounding alveolar bone.[40] The pathogens responsible for the inflammation originate in the pulp cavity, but the inflammatory process that creates the granuloma originates in the periodontium. For the purpose of classification, the apical granuloma is a periodontal lesion of endodontic origin.

Fig 2-1 *(a to e)* Periodontal lesions of endodontic origin at the apex *(red circles and arrow)*.

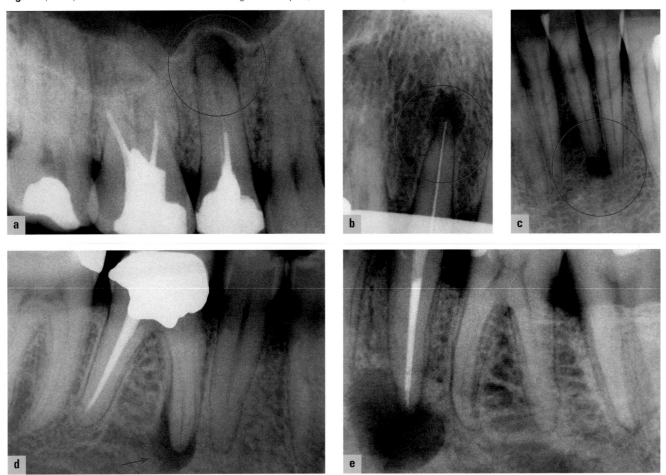

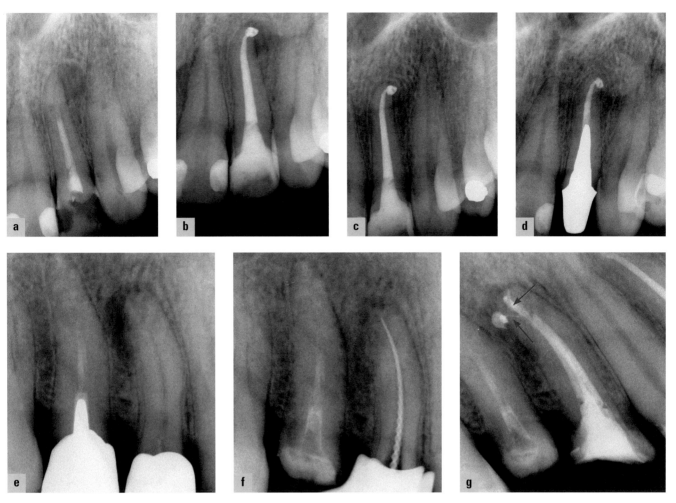

Fig 2-2 *(a to g)* Periodontal lesions of endodontic origin extending apicolaterally.

Fig 2-3 *(a to c)* Periodontal lesions of endodontic origin along the lateral root surface.

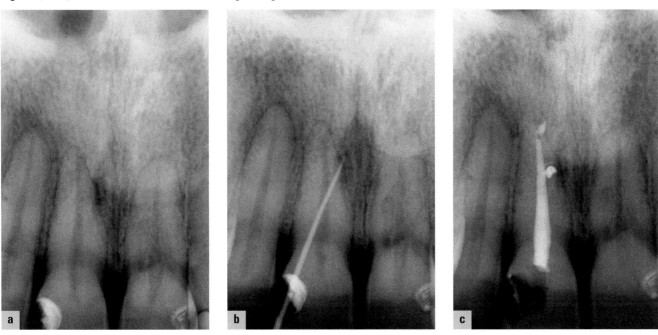

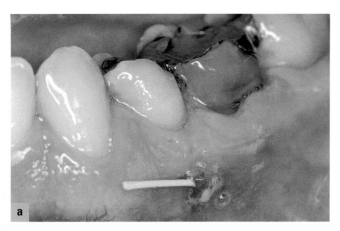 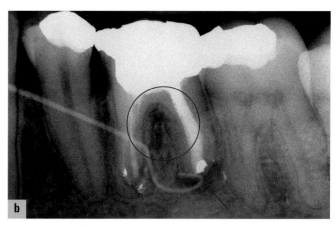

Figs 2-4a and 2-4b　Periodontal lesion of endodontic origin affecting a mandibular left first molar. A sinus tract is located mesiobuccal to the affected molar. Radiolucencies are located apically *(arrow)* and interradicularly *(circle)*. The radiograph also indicates the probable point of origin of the lesion, the apex of the distal root. The tooth has been previously treated with an apicoectomy and is symptomatic again.

Figs 2-4c to 2-4h　The apicoectomy failed as a result of step-back obturation performed on an improperly cleansed endodontic substrate. Note caries underneath the amalgam restoration. The treatment plan involved thorough removal of caries and infected tissue, endodontic retreatment, and restoration with a metal-ceramic crown. *(f)* The gutta-percha filling has ejected the apical amalgam of the original apicoectomy.

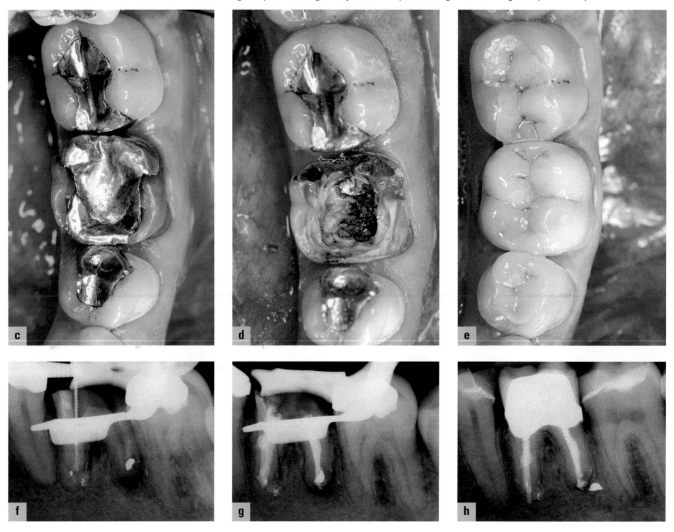

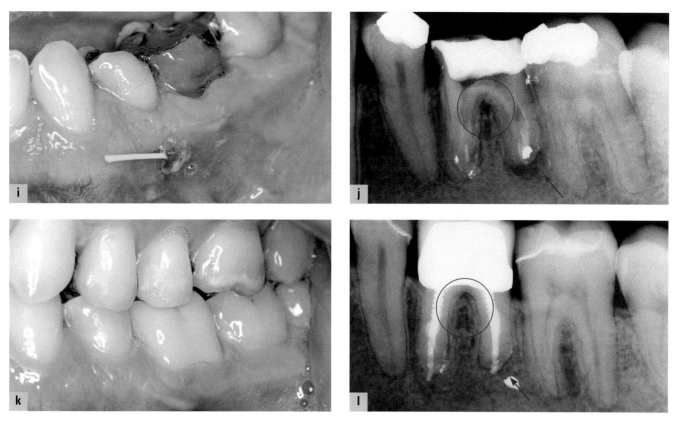

Figs 2-4i to 2-4l The mandibular left first molar seen pretreatment *(i and j)* and 6 years posttreatment *(k and l)*.

Figs 2-4m to 2-4p Soft tissue and osseous contours 10 years posttreatment.

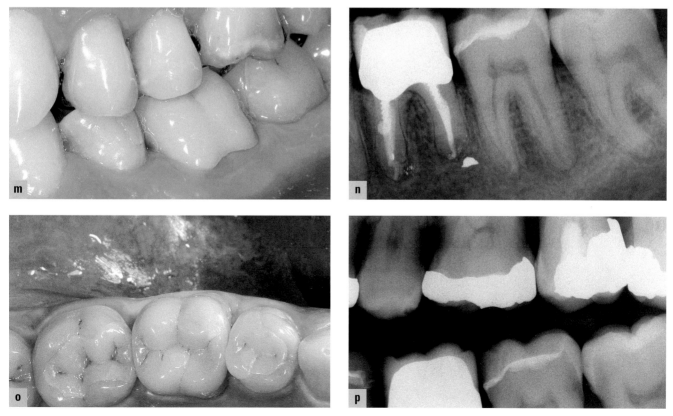

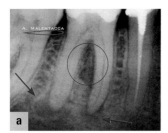 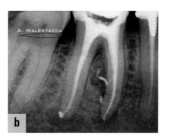 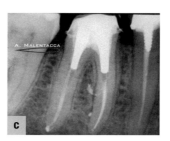 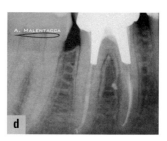

Fig 2-5 *(a to d)* The mandibular right first molar presented with apical *(red circle)* and interradicular radiolucency *(red arrows)*. The absence of periodontal pockets, a negative response to vitality testing, and the sizable restoration reflected the endodontic nature of the pathology. The successful outcome following endodontic treatment confirmed the accuracy of the initial diagnosis. (Courtesy of Dr Augusto Malentacca.)

Fig 2-6 *(a and b)* Lesions of endodontic origin affecting the apical, periradicular, and interradicular periodontium. Healing following root canal treatment confirmed the diagnosis. (Courtesy of Dr Fabio Gorni.)

Fig 2-7 *(a and b)* A canal opening into the pulp cavity floor.

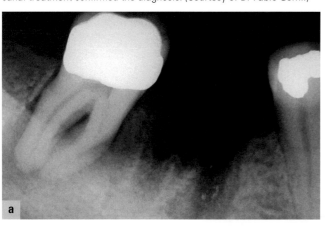 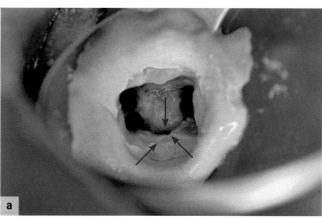

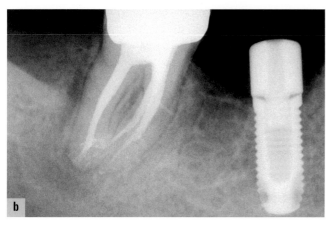 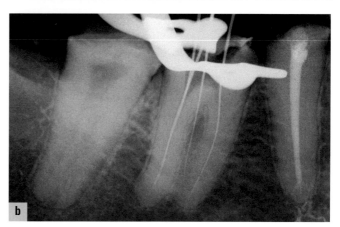

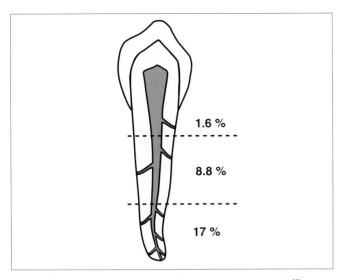

Fig 2-8 Prevalence of lateral canals decrease apicomarginally.[37]

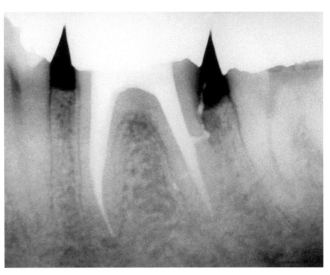

Fig 2-9 The distal root of a mandibular left first molar has a lateral canal that has created a periodontal lesion of endodontic origin. A probing depth of 6 mm was recorded at this surface; probing depth was 3 mm at other surfaces. This lesion of periodontal attachment could have been easily mistaken for a plaque-induced periodontitis. Observe another lateral canal on the mesial aspect of the distal root, near the middle third. (Courtesy of Dr Fabio Gorni.)

Fig 2-10 *(a)* The maxillary left central incisor presented with an angular bony defect in the middle third of the mesial surface. Vitality testing was inconclusive. *(b)* Endodontic treatment revealed a lateral canal at the same height as the bony defect. *(c)* A 4-month posttreatment radiograph shows that the defect has healed completely. (Courtesy of Prof Elio Berutti, Turin, Italy.)

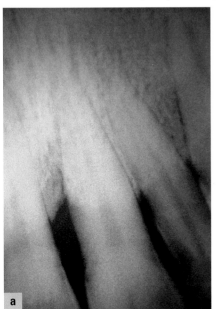

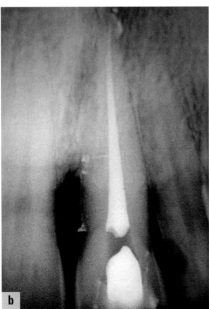

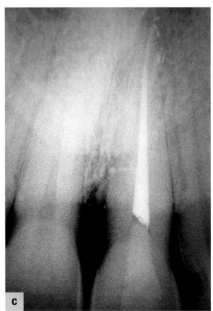

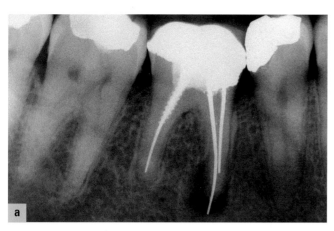 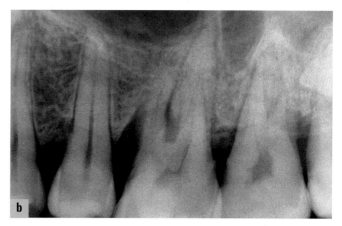

Fig 2-11 Lesions seen in their classical presentations. *(a)* An apically situated periodontal lesion of endodontic origin. *(b)* A bony defect from chronic periodontitis.

Fig 2-12 *(a to d)* Teeth with both endodontic pathology and bony defects from chronic periodontitis.

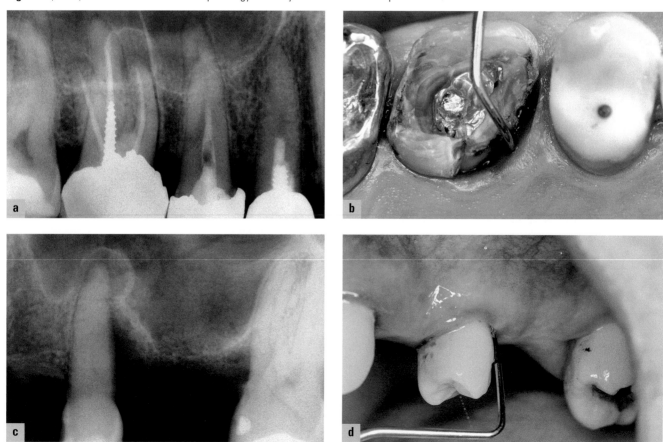

Plaque-Induced Periodontal Lesions

Periodontitis is inflammation of the supporting tissues surrounding the tooth and extends from gingiva into the adjacent bone and periodontal ligament. It results in loss of attachment and pocket formation. The most common cause is plaque and dental calculus, and the most common diagnosis is chronic periodontitis. Plaque-induced periodontitis can also lead to abscess formation.

Differential Diagnosis

Plaque-induced periodontal lesions and periodontal lesions of endodontic origin may share radiologic and clinical symptoms. Effective treatment is dependent upon the clinician's ability to distinguish among them. The location of the pathology is the first thing to consider when starting the differential diagnosis. A periodontitis of endodontic origin will likely present symptoms associated with the apical third of the root whereas a plaque-related periodontitis will typically involve the coronal third of the root (Fig 2-11). The following are potential symptoms of both general classifications:
- Inflammation of the gingival margin
- Increased tooth mobility
- Sensitivity to percussion and/or pressure
- Blood or purulent exudate
- Increased probing depth[41]

A more challenging case for the diagnostician is the tooth that presents with mixed pathology, originating both internally in the canal and externally from the periodontium (Fig 2-12). Radiographs may show a tooth with concurrent periradicular and periapical radiolucency (Figs 2-13 and 2-14). It is essential to understand fully the interrelationship between pathologic processes of endodontic origin and those of periodontal origin. When symptoms have overlapping features, this understanding is necessary to establish the exact etiopathogenesis of the lesion, which is the starting point for a correct treatment plan.[42] Subsequent chapters will elaborate on classification and diagnosis of both types of lesion.

Clinical Cases

Two complex cases (Figs 2-15 and 2-16) illustrate the importance of diagnosing and treating plaque-induced periodontal disease separately from periodontal lesions of pulpal origin.   ■

Fig 2-13 *(a and b)* Radiographs show lesions simultaneously affecting both apical and marginal areas.

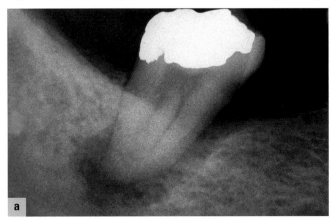
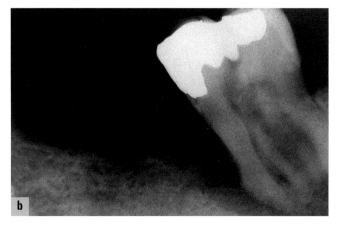

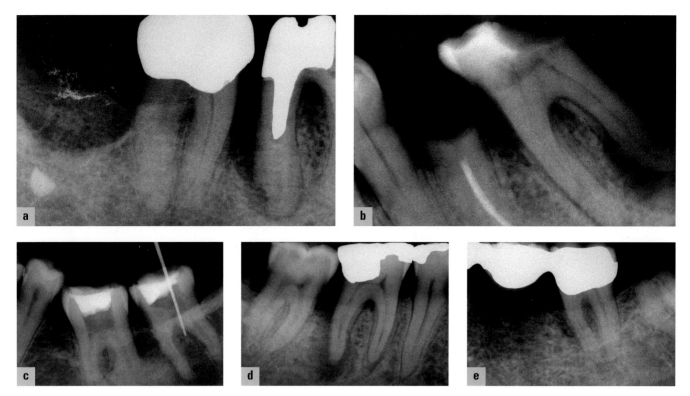

Fig 2-14 *(a to e)* Further lesions simultaneously affecting both apical and marginal areas.

61-year-old male patient

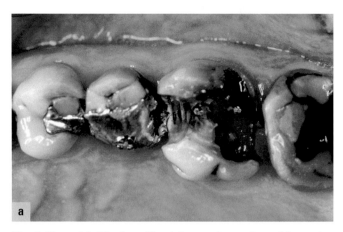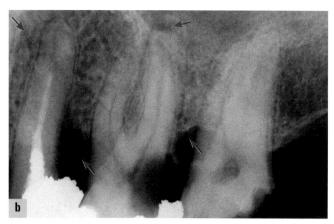

Figs 2-15a and 2-15b A maxillary left second premolar and first molar are affected by periodontal lesions of endodontic origin and plaque-induced periodontal disease.

Figs 2-15c to 2-15k The treatment plan called for endodontic tooth rehabilitation. *(d)* Note the three canals in the mesiobuccal root of the molar.

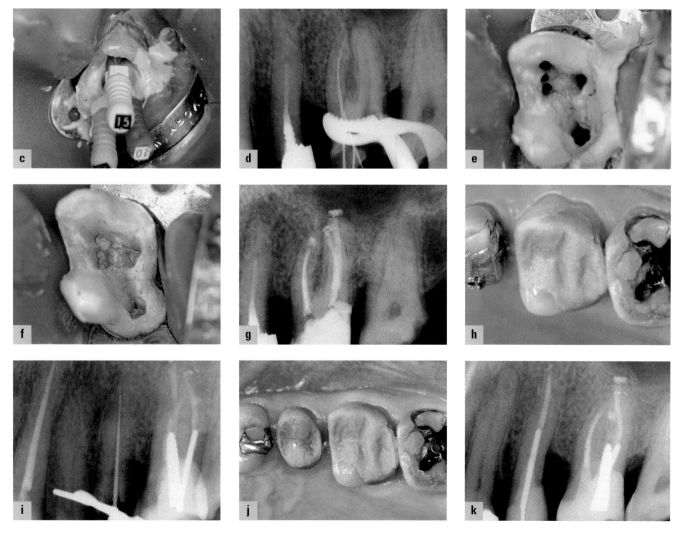

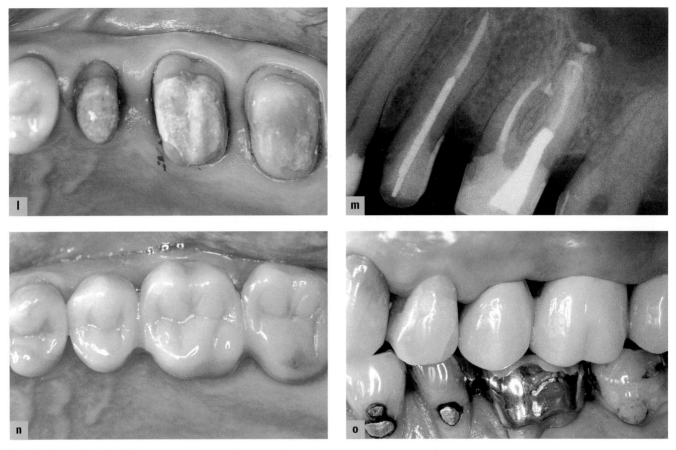

Figs 2-15l to 2-15o   Preliminary core preparation *(l and m)* and provisional restorations *(n and o).*

Figs 2-15p to 2-15u   *(p to r)* In order to eliminate the periodontal defects[43] and restore correct tissue architecture,[44,45] osseous resective surgery was performed,[46] conserving the gingival fibers.[47,48] Core preparation was completed intraoperatively.[49,50] *(s to u)* After healing, the case was completed with a ceramic inlay on the first premolar, metal-ceramic crowns on the second premolar and first molar, and a gold crown on the second molar.

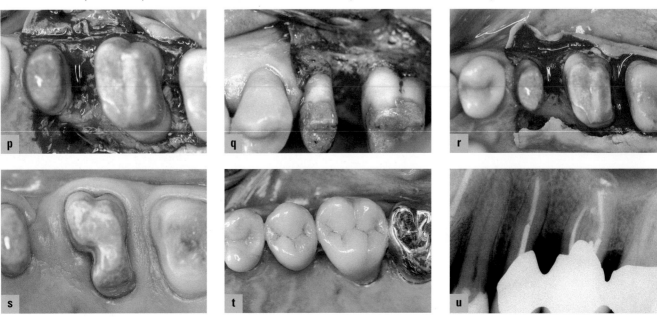

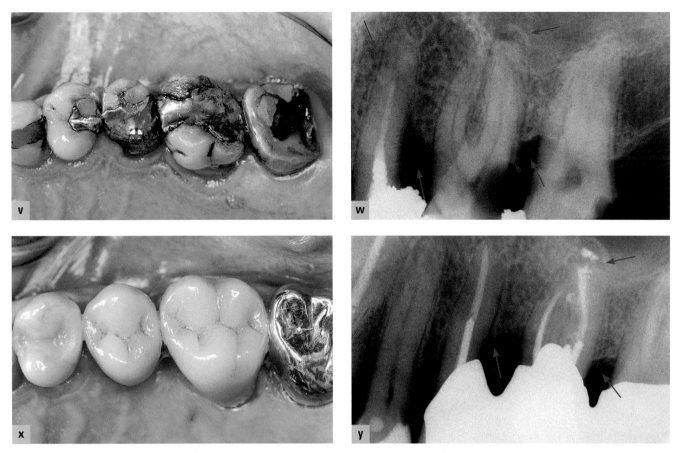

Figs 2-15v to 2-15y Pretreatment *(v and w)* and 2-year posttreatment records *(x and y)* showing lack of inflammation, physiologic bony contours, and apical healing *(arrows)*.

Figs 2-15z and 2-15aa After 9 years, all periodontal lesions, both those of endodontic origin and plaque-induced, have healed and show no sign of returning.

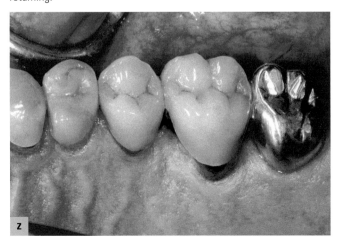

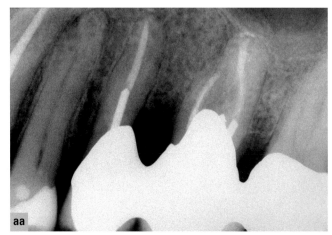

40-year-old female patient

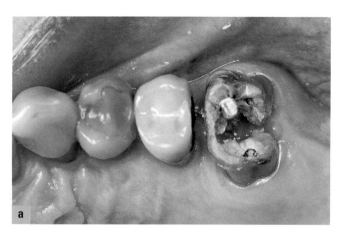 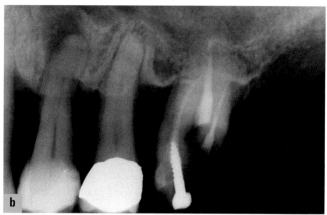

Figs 2-16a and 2-16b Chronic periodontitis and apical periodontitis in the maxillary left posterior.

Figs 2-16c to 2-16f Clinical photographs and radiographs show the poor prognosis and limited treatment options for this patient's dentition.

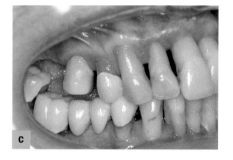 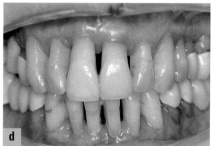 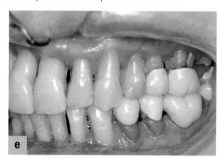

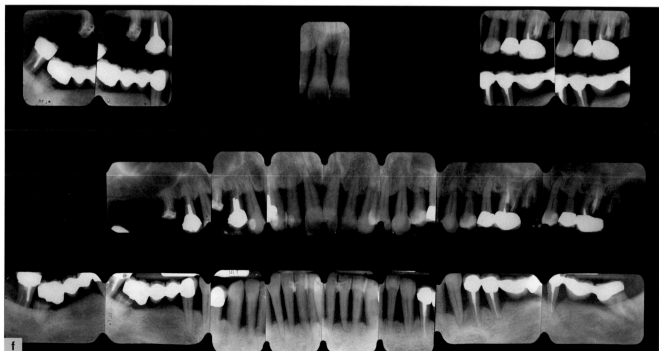

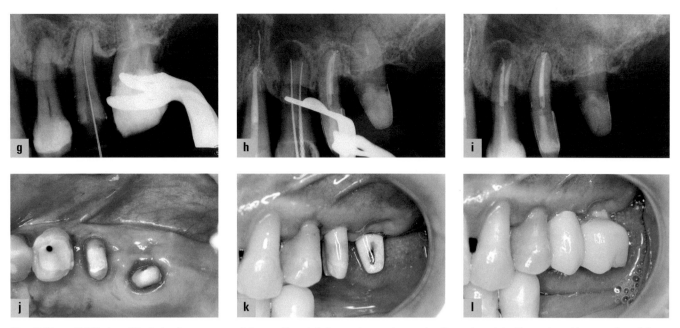

Figs 2-16g to 2-16l *(g to i)* Endodontic treatment of the maxillary left first and second premolar. Resection of the first molar with extraction of the buccal roots and endodontic treatment of the remaining palatal root. *(j to l)* Post and core preparation and provisional restorations.

Figs 2-16m to 2-16r Surgical treatment of plaque-induced periodontal disease. Flaps trimmed prior to osseous resective surgery[46] conserving the gingival fibers.[47,48] Intraoperative core preparation[49,50] using burs nos. 6862 and 8862 (Komet) and fitting of new provisional restorations.

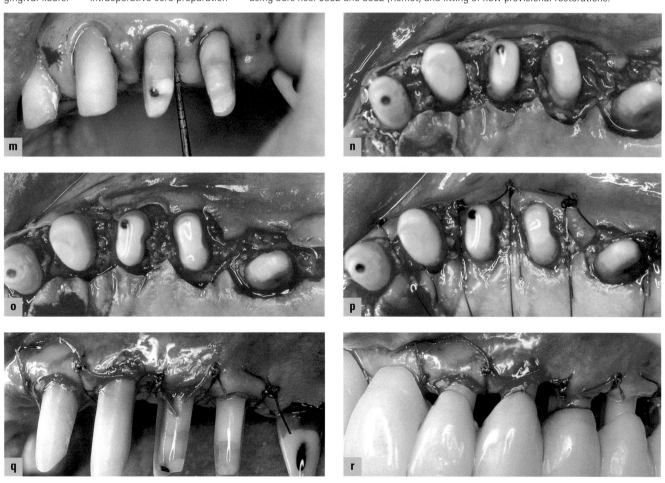

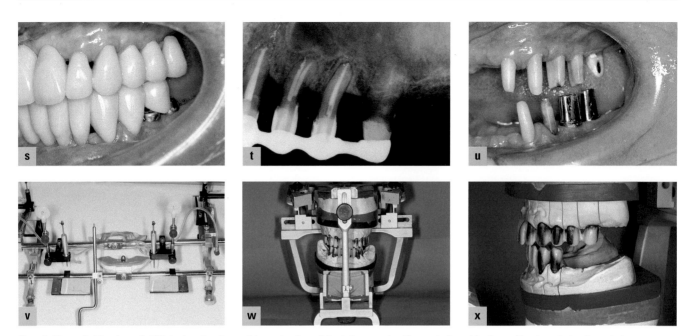

Figs 2-16s to 2-16x *(s and t)* Clinical and radiographic evaluation of the left posterior. The periodontal lesions of both endodontic and plaque-induced origin have been treated and have healed. *(u)* Final impression stage. *(v to x)* Facebow recording, customized articulator mounting, and initial wax-up of restorations.

Figs 2-16y to 2-16bb Completed case. (Prosthodontics courtesy of Dr Gianfranco di Febo, and Mr Roberto Bonfiglioli.)

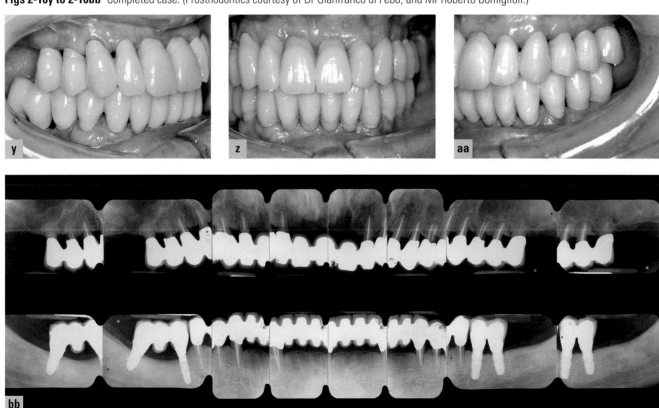

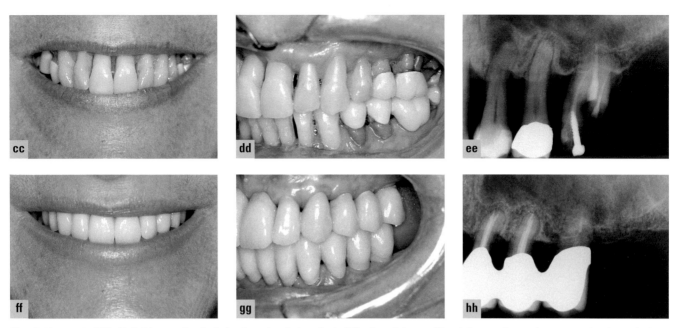

Figs 2-16cc to 2-16hh Definitive results. Endodontic and periodontal rehabilitation of the maxillary left posterior quadrant was a key factor in the overall outcome and maintenance of the patient's smile.

Figs 2-16ii to 2-16ll Restorations and soft tissue contours 1 year *(ii and jj)* and 3 years *(kk and ll)* after final cementation.

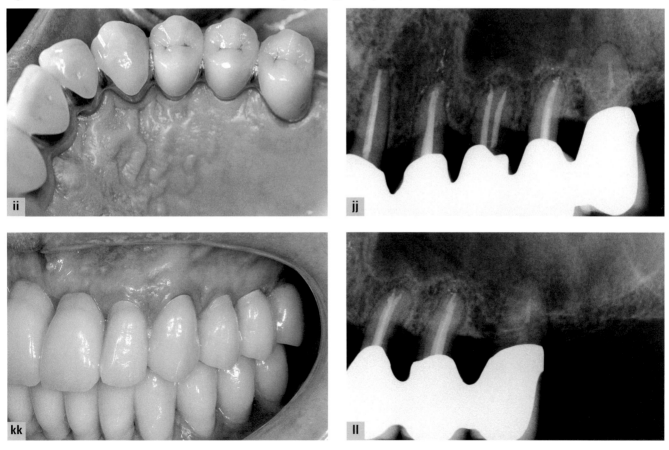

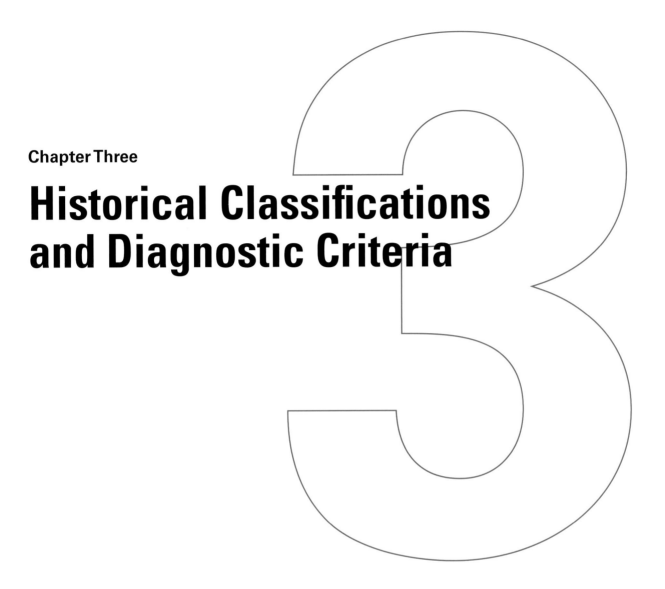

Chapter Three

Historical Classifications and Diagnostic Criteria

In 1972 Simon, Glick and Frank[2] proposed a classification system based on the etiopathogenesis of tooth-support–apparatus lesions with reference to their endodontic and periodontal origins. The classification system includes five distinct categories:

1. Primary endodontic lesion
2. Primary endodontic lesion with secondary periodontal involvement
3. Primary periodontal lesion
4. Primary periodontal lesion with secondary endodontic involvement
5. True combined lesions

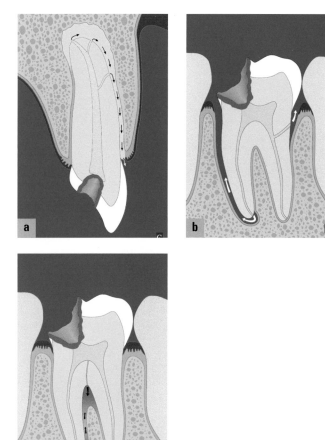

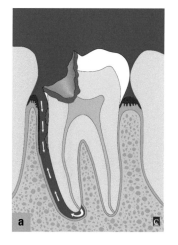

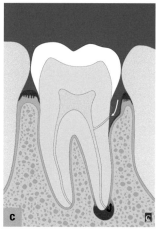

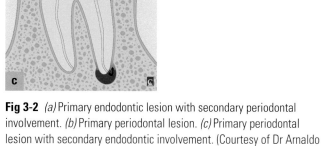

Fig 3-1 Primary endodontic lesions with suppurative drainage via: apical *(a)*, lateral *(b)*, and accessory foramina *(c)*. (Courtesy of Dr Arnaldo Castellucci.)

Fig 3-2 *(a)* Primary endodontic lesion with secondary periodontal involvement. *(b)* Primary periodontal lesion. *(c)* Primary periodontal lesion with secondary endodontic involvement. (Courtesy of Dr Arnaldo Castellucci.)

Fig 3-3 Combined endo-perio lesions, merging *(a)* and separate *(b)*. (Courtesy of Dr Arnaldo Castellucci.)

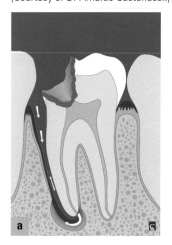

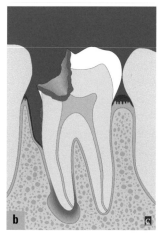

Primary Endodontic Lesions

Suppurative matter created by endodontic pathology can drain externally through the periodontal ligament in a sinus tract that terminates in the gingival sulcus. The affected tooth permits probing of considerable depth, the cause of which requires investigation. Where it has been ascertained that the tooth has necrotized pulp (as confirmed by negative vitality tests, including cavity testing as a last resort) and a suspected apical or pararadicular lesion is indicated by radiograph, probing of the sulcus will reveal a deep narrow defect. This tube-like defect will extend as far as the apex or the point of the root where a lateral canal emerges, according to the source of infection (Fig 3-1).

Primary Endodontic Lesions with Secondary Periodontal Involvement

These lesions are a common development of the previous class of lesion. The continuing presence of the sulcular orifice of a sinus tract as a consequence of untreated or unsuccessfully treated endodontic pathology permits infiltration of bacteria from plaque or calculus that colonize the root surface along the sinus tract path. The result is loss of attachment and apical migration of the junctional epithelium (Fig 3-2a).

Primary Periodontal Lesions

Chronic periodontal disease, with its accumulation of plaque and calculus, will progress apically if not arrested by appropriate treatment (Fig 3-2b). Pulp testing will reveal a vital pulp. Upon probing, pocket configuration will typically be broader and pockets more generalized throughout the dentition than in cases of primary endodontic lesions.

Primary Periodontal Lesions with Secondary Endodontic Involvement

Simon, Glick and Frank[2] describe this classification as a potential development of primary periodontal lesions. As destruction of the attachment apparatus progresses apically, lateral or accessory canals may become exposed to periodontal pathogens that lead to retrograde pulp necrosis (Fig 3-2c). Other authors maintain that this situation is theoretically possible but not easily confirmed clinically.[51–53]

Combined Lesions

Two independent pathologies may coexist in the same tooth (Fig 3-3a). Endodontic disease progressing coronally and a periodontal pocket advancing apically may meet and merge.

Dr Arnaldo Castellucci has addressed this classification and suggests limiting the definition of combined lesion to situations in which the two pathologies have yet to come into communication with one another and are still distinct (Fig 3-3b).[6]

New Diagnostic Criteria for Endo-Perio Lesions

Although feasible and didactically interesting, the above classifications add little to prevailing analysis of endo-perio conditions. The two clinical cases cited in chapter 2 (see Figs 2-15 and 2-16) present typical situations in which the periodontium is affected simultaneously by two distinct pathologies, usually a combination of plaque-induced periodontal disease and an apical endodontic lesion.

Immediate, straightforward identification of lesions on the basis of location and a set of signs and symptoms is not compatible with a true differential diagnosis, which is essential in dealing with endo-perio patients.

Imagine applying a simple screening approach based on two key points: (1) Does the tooth have a lesion? (2) If so, is the lesion endodontic or periodontal?

Although every clinical detail must be considered in the event that it could tip the balance towards one diagnosis or another, two data should be given priority:

1. *Periodontal probing.* Depth and pocket configuration can provide essential information into the nature of the lesion causing the pockets. In the absence of significant pockets, plaque-induced periodontal disease can be ruled out.
2. *Pulp vitality testing.* Results indicating a vital pulp categorically exclude a periodontal lesion of endodontic origin. When findings point to pulp necrosis or are dubious, probing should be revisited.

Bear in mind that significant pocket depths can be associated with:

- Sinus tract due to a periodontal lesion of endodontic origin
- Attachment loss due to a plaque-related periodontal condition
- Coexistence of both conditions, in which case the cause and extent of each lesion must be established (Fig 3-4)

The term *endo-perio* lesion describes a clinical situation and poses a diagnostic query. Once the presence of both endodontic and periodontal symptoms has been ascertained, the term alone has no further helpful meaning and more diagnostically relevant terms are needed. While a landmark text in its day, the classifications of Simon, Glick, and Frank should now be finessed from a clinical and practical point of view into a clearer diagnostic tool.

The time has come to propose an alternative classification system based on observation of clinical situations. These are summarized in chapter 4 according to their logical sequence.

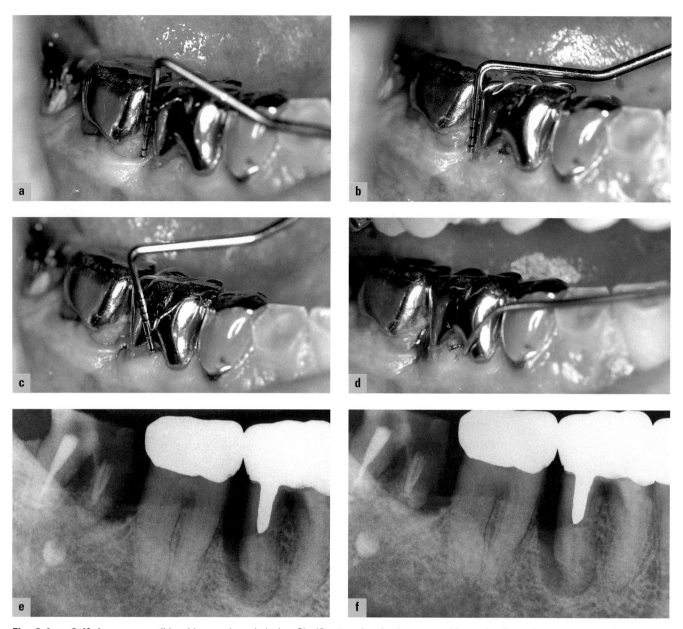

Figs 3-4a to 3-4f A case compatible with an endo-perio lesion. Significant pocket depths upon probing and radiographs show advanced attachment loss at the mesial surface of the lower right mandibular third molar and the distal surface of the nearby first molar. The interradicular areas of both teeth also have attachment loss.

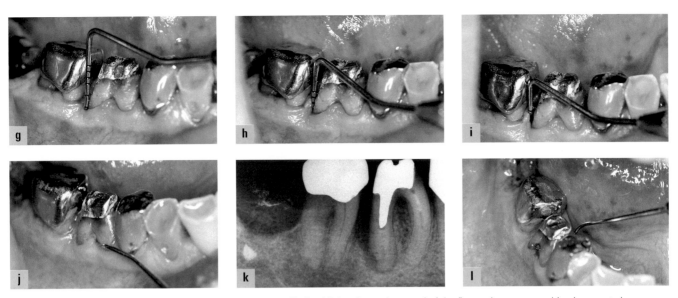

Figs 3-4g to 3-4l Following extraction of the lower right mandibular third molar and removal of the first molar crown, probing is repeated. Presumed diagnosis is combined endo-perio lesion.

Figs 3-4m and 3-4n With the probe in place, a radiograph confirms the apical extent of the defect.

Fig 3-4o Post removed prior to endodontic treatment.

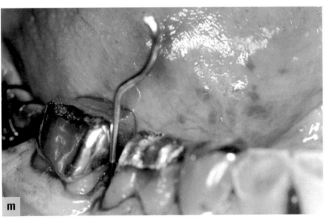

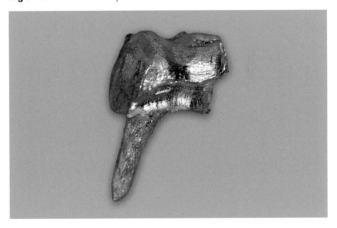

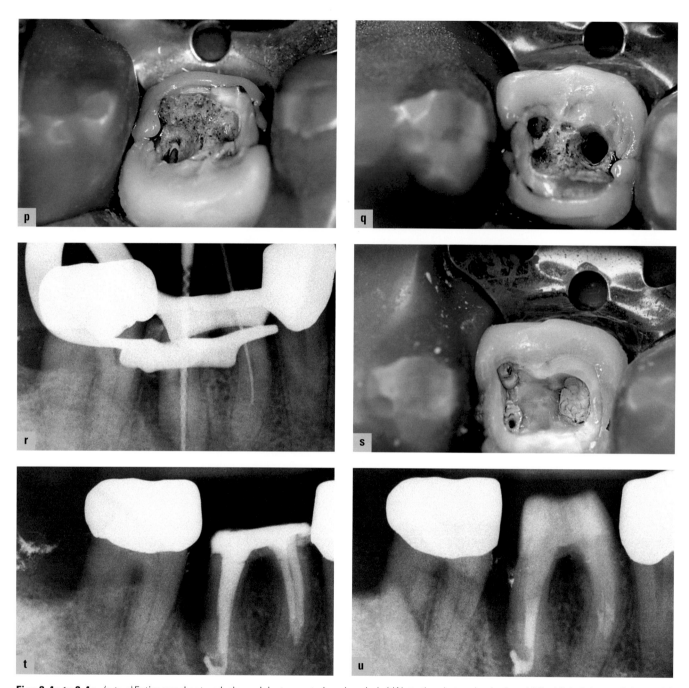

Figs 3-4p to 3-4u *(p to s)* Entire canal network cleaned, instrumented, and sealed. *(t)* Note the obstruction in the middle third of the mesial root. *(u)* The point of obstruction dictated the working length of this canal rather than risking harmful over-instrumentation.

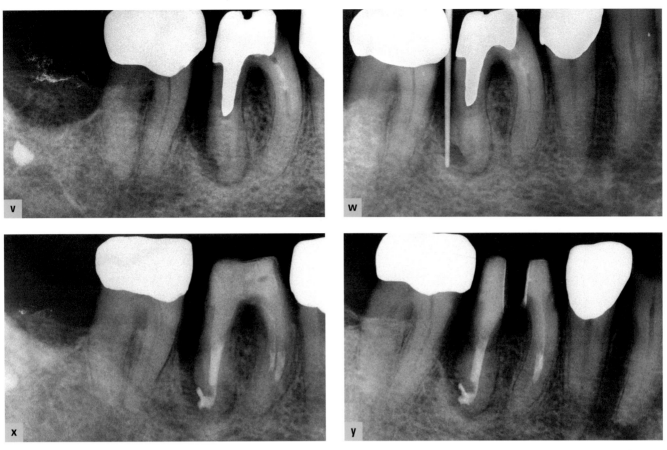

Figs 3-4v to 3-4y Pretreatment radiograph *(v)* and 3-month *(x)* and 6-month *(y)* radiographs following endodontic treatment. After the 3-month follow-up, the patient underwent scaling and root planing followed by hemisection of the first molar. Once the endodontic source of the periodontal lesion was successfully treated and the plaque and infected cementum eliminated, the situation improved both objectively and subjectively. Probing depth remained at 5 mm with no inflammation. Since the patient is asymptomatic and aged 85, the decision was made to accept the 5-mm pocket depth and to continue to monitor the situation.

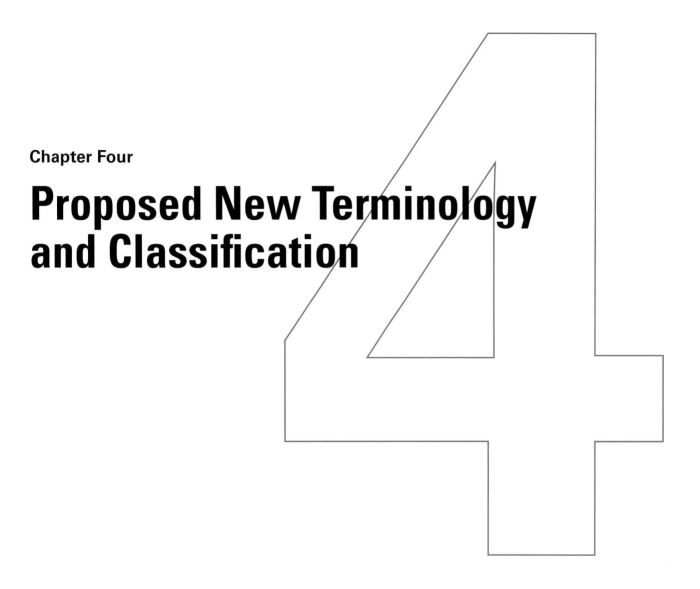

Chapter Four
Proposed New Terminology and Classification

The expression *endo-perio lesion* is commonly used[2–6]; it is concise and at the same time encompasses many pathologies; however, as with many conveniences, the term *endo-perio* lacks the level of specificity required for clinical usefulness. New nomenclature is needed that is both brief and adequately descriptive of the pathological progression of the two general categories discussed in chapter 2.

Endo-perio lesions will now be divided into three categories[1] rather than the five proposed by Simon, Glick, and Frank.[2]

- Class 1: Crown-down plaque-induced periodontal lesions
- Class 2: Down-crown periodontal lesions of endodontic origin
- Class 3: Combined endo-perio lesions

A fourth, interim classification is useful for the purpose of diagnosis: *pseudo endo-perio lesions*, for situations in which the initial clinical and radiologic examination points to both endodontic and periodontal sources. Pulp vitality, or lack thereof, and the results of periodontal probing resolve diagnostic doubt concerning a lesion's true nature, which is then definitively identified as Class 1, 2, or 3. Case studies in chapter 5 will expand on this topic.

Diagnosis of Crown-Down and Down-Crown Lesions

The cornerstones of diagnosing, classifying, and treating this pathology are periodontal probing and pulp vitality testing, supported by analysis of radiographs. So long as these lesions remain confined to their respective areas of origin, their position alone is often sufficient to determine their true nature (see Fig 2-13). However, as they progress, diagnosis may become more elusive.

Probing as a diagnostic tool

If probing depths are abnormal at a number of points within the same gingival sulcus, a diagnosis of crown-down plaque-induced periodontal lesion is plausible. Positive vitality testing in such cases will rule out any endodontic involvement.

On the other hand, deep marginal probing does not necessarily correspond to attachment loss and consequent apical migration of the junctional epithelium. The probe may locate the path of a sinus tract running through the periodontal ligament (PDL), the result of endodontic pathology (Figs 4-1 and 4-2). In such cases, the suppurating cavity has created a drainage path according to the principle of locus minoris resistentiae (the path of least resistance). The sinus tract is therefore a pathway by which the body reduces the pressure and pathogen load within a closed space, with the root apex or a lateral canal serving as the source of infection. Therefore, an isolated, tube-like area of probe penetration (Fig 4-2) indicates a sinus tract draining an endodontic lesion secondary to a cause such as vertical root fracture (Figs 4-3 and 4-4). Probing should be correlated with radiographs of the tooth being examined.

Fig 4-1 *(a)* Periodontal probing of the maxillary right second premolar follows the path of a sinus tract draining intrasulcularly from an apically located endodontic lesion. *(b)* Surgical endodontic treatment. (Courtesy of Dr Fabio Gorni.)

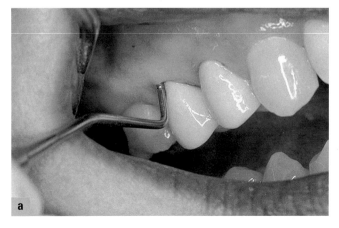
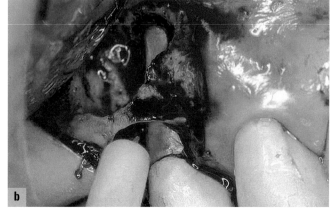

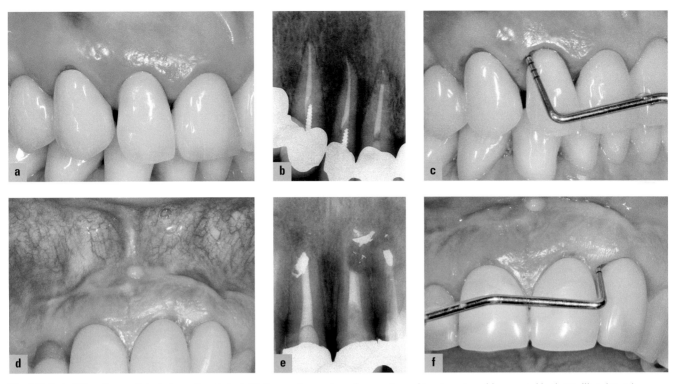

Fig 4-2 *(a to f)* Despite no clinical signs of periodontal inflammation and previous root canal treatment, probing around both maxillary lateral incisors locates narrow pockets consistent with draining sinus tracts.

Fig 4-3 Maxillary right lateral incisor. *(a)* Access flap for diagnostic purposes. *(b)* Exposure of the root surface revealing vertical fracture line. *(c and d)* Extraction.

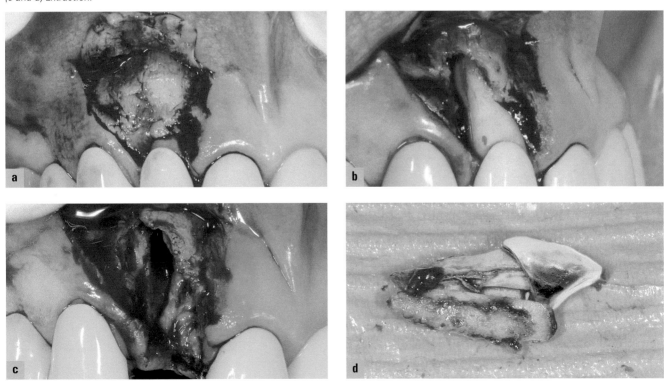

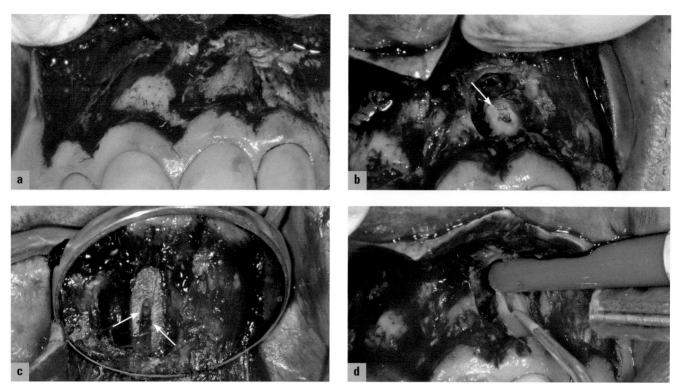

Figs 4-4a to 4-4d Maxillary left lateral incisor. *(a)* Scalloped perimarginal incision and creation of a total thickness access flap. *(b)* Exposure of root apex shows apicoectomy amalgam filling and fracture line extending mesiopalatally *(arrow)*. *(c)* Retrograde cavity preparation *(arrows)* has damaged the root well beyond the natural canal. *(d)* Amalgam removed, canal sterilized, and fracture line smoothed prior to use of ultrasound tips (ProUltra, Maillefer) for retrograde cavity preparation along true canal path.

Figs 4-4e to 4-4i *(e and f)* Retrograde sealing with mineral trioxide aggregate (ProRoot MTA [Maillefer]) of the left lateral incisor and both central incisors. 5-0 Vicryl sutures (Ethicon) *(g)* and postoperative control radiographs *(h and i)*.

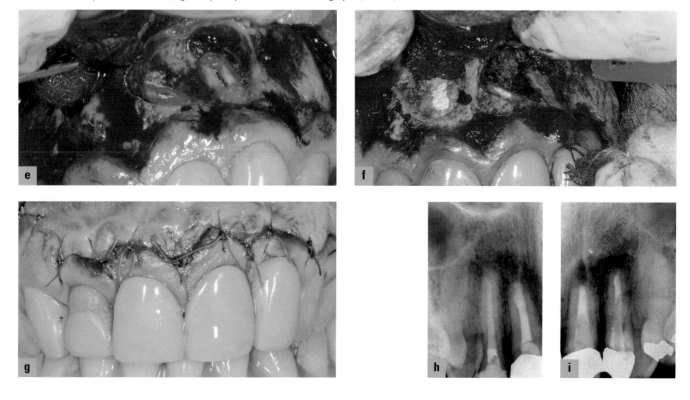

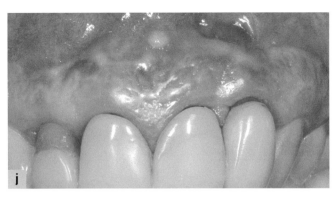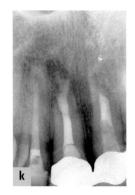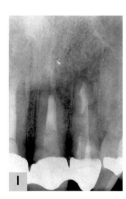

Figs 4-4j to 4-4l Healthy tissues and bone regrowth 6 months postoperation.

A sinus tract draining intrasulcularly may reach this position by two routes (Figs 4-5 and 4-6).

1. Exudate originating from a periapical abscess burrows its way towards the crown through the fibers of the PDL parallel to the tooth (Fig 4-6a). The sinus tract created in the PDL space can be inspected with a probe or gutta-percha point. The probe as it forces its way towards the gingival margin, penetrates a web of tissue stretched by the suppurating matter (Fig 4-6b).
2. Exudate reaches the surface along a subperiosteal route, traveling first perpendicularly through the alveolar bone (Fig 4-5b). This process is named *extraosseous-subperiosteal fistulization*, and it tends to develop on the buccal surface where tissues are thinner. It is not likely to result in misleading findings upon probing.

Sinus tracts commonly present intraoral draining at a point close to their origin, generally through the buccal or lingual mucosa of the infected tooth. They may also exit at a more remote point, often through the buccal mucosa of an adjacent tooth[54,55] (Figs 4-7 to 4-9). Sinus tracts draining through the gingival sulcus (creating a narrow defect) usually do so at the involved tooth but may also drain through the sulcus of an adjacent tooth (Figs 4-10 to 4-13).

Because of the existence of dual causes for similar probing results, it is necessary to ascertain the true cause of all pockets and to always chart probing readings carefully. Probing takes on greater significance when the patient has teeth with potential or confirmed endodontic lesions, a history of trauma, orthodontic treatment,[16,56] episodes of pain, extensive or deep fillings, or changes in tooth color.[14,57]

In summary, narrow, isolated pockets are associated with down-crown lesions of endodontic origin. Broader pockets, often found at multiple points on a single tooth, are associated with crown-down plaque-induced periodontal lesions.

Fig 4-5 *(a)* Dental-periodontium apparatus. *(b)* Probing of a pocket with loss of attachment. *(c)* Probing of the PDL space with attachment apparatus intact, though altered by exudate and inflammatory products.

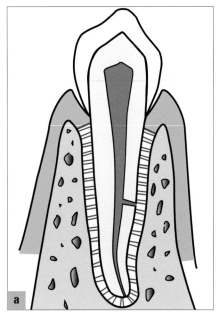
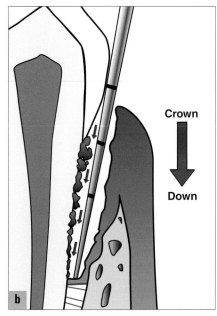
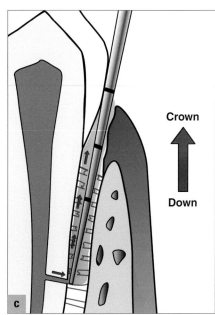

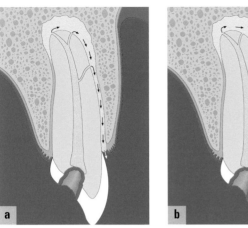

Fig 4-6 *(a)* Intrasulcular drainage through the PDL space. *(b)* Intrasulcular drainage through a subperiosteal route. (Courtesy of Dr Arnaldo Castellucci.)

Fig 4-7 *(a)* Draining sinus tract near maxillary right second premolar previously treated with root canal therapy (RCT) and restored with a metal-ceramic crown. *(b)* Radiograph shows evidence of marginal leakage. *(c and d)* A gutta-percha point inserted into the tract follows it to the apex of the first premolar, where an area of apical radiolucency indicates a lesion of endodontic origin.

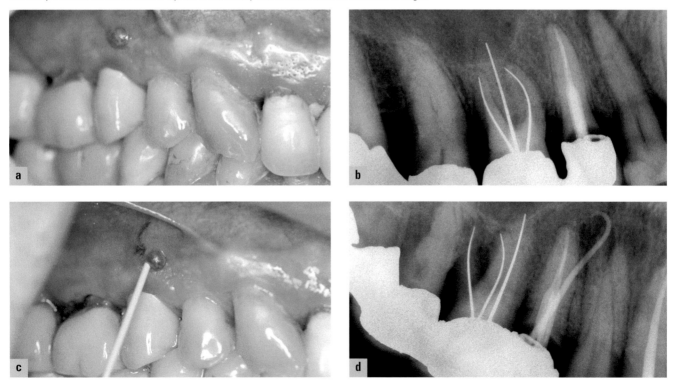

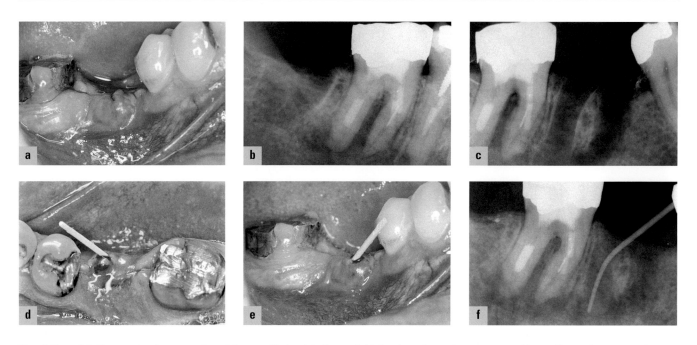

Figs 4-8a to 4-f Two weeks after extraction of the mandibular right first and third molars, the patient presents with swelling and presence of a draining tract whose pathway appears to originate from the distal aspect of the first molar extraction site. Clinical evaluation and radiographs suggest osteomyelitis rather than a retained root fragment. However, the second molar adjacent to the sinus tract has inadequate root canal obturation and periapical radiolucency, indicating a more likely cause of the ensuing pus drainage.

Figs 4-8g to 4-8k Stages of endodontic retreatment. The apical foramen has been altered by previous instrumentation and resorption, hindering satisfactory control of sealants, especially in the mesiobuccal canal.

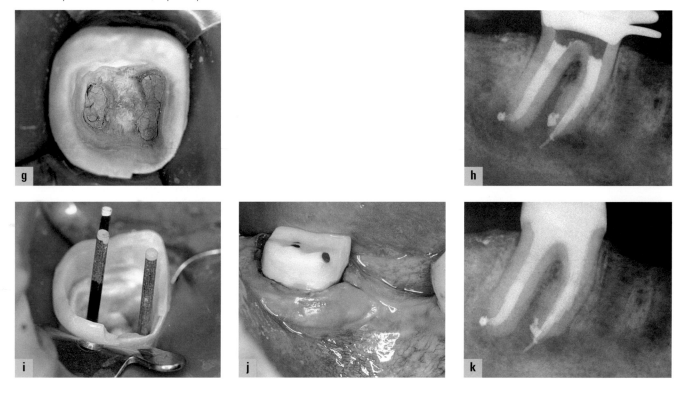

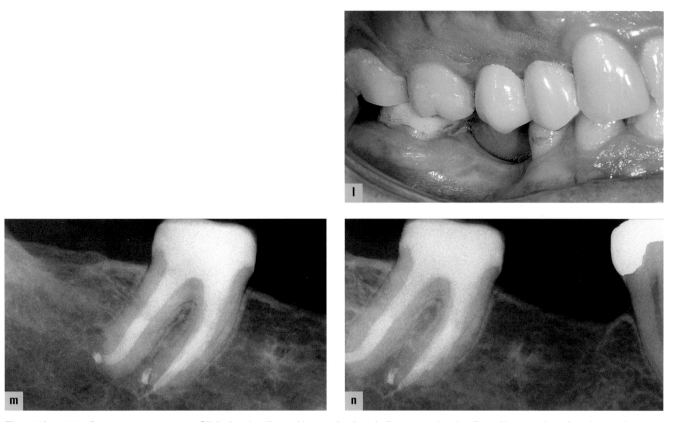

Figs 4-8l to 4-8n One year posttreatment. Clinical and radiographic examinations indicate complete healing with resorption of much extruded sealant. For financial reasons, the patient declined surgical prosthodontic rehabilitation.

Figs 4-9a to 4-9d *(a)* Swelling in the area of a fixed partial denture (FPD) in the maxillary left quadrant. *(b)* Radiograph showed endodontically treated teeth with no visible apical changes. *(d)* Flossing under the FPD removed plaque and debris and caused copious bleeding. It was concluded that plaque accumulation below the pontic had caused the inflammation.

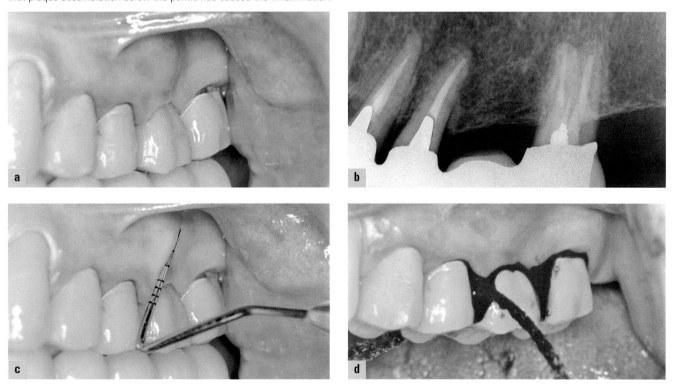

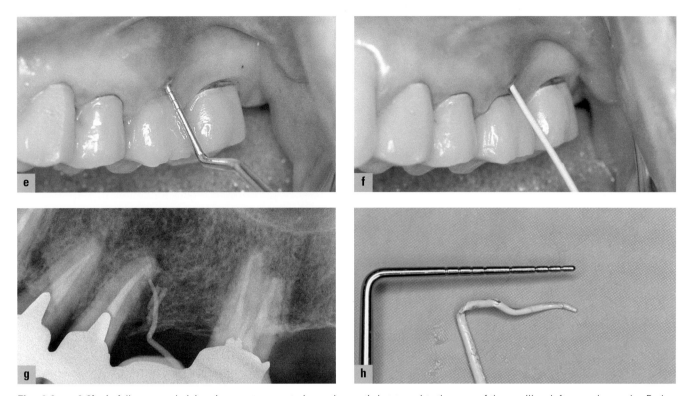

Figs 4-9e to 4-9h At follow-up, a draining sinus tract was noted near the pontic but traced to the apex of the maxillary left second premolar. Both premolars were found to be fractured and were extracted.

Fig 4-10 *(a)* The patient presented with swelling facial to the maxillary left lateral incisor and canine following fracture and debonding of an FPD. In spite of generalized periodontal health, there were two deep pockets greater than 10 mm around these two teeth. *(b and c)* A lesion of endodontic origin at the apex of the lateral incisor had created two drainage routes along the PDL spaces of the lateral incisor and canine. *(d and e)* Endodontic treatment of the lateral incisor resulted in healing of both sites. An error of diagnosis and ensuing periodontal treatment such as scaling and root planing could have caused irreversible damage.

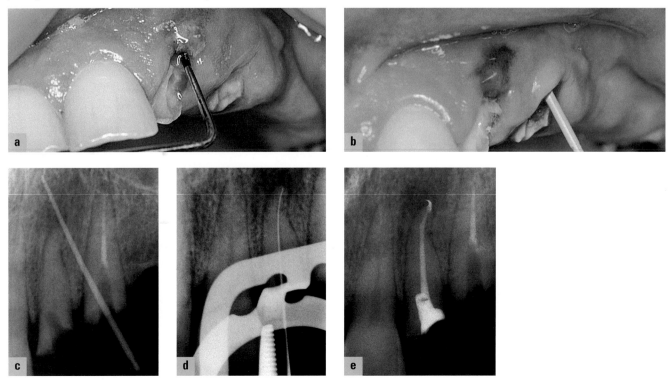

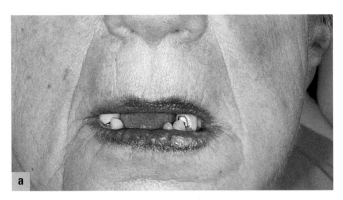

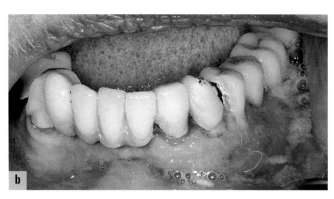

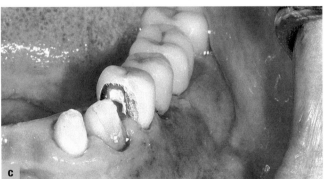

Figs 4-11a to 4-11c A 73-year-old patient presented with significant swelling on the lower left. Examination revealed vestibular swelling and copious purulent exudate at the marginal gingiva in the mandibular left posterior. An anterior FPD had debonded and was removed. The underlying abutment teeth were found to be stable.

Figs 4-11d to 4-11f Periodontal probing located a significant pocket on the facial surface of the canine abutment. A gutta-percha cone inserted into the pocket extended past the canine apex and continued toward the alveolar nerve foramen.

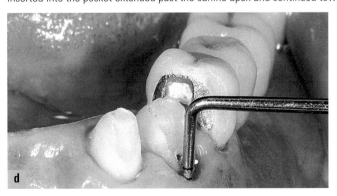

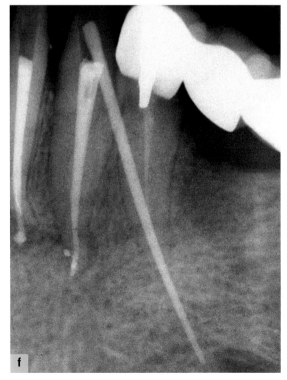

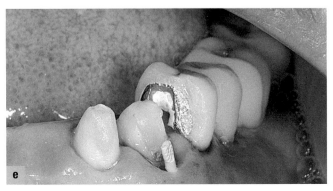

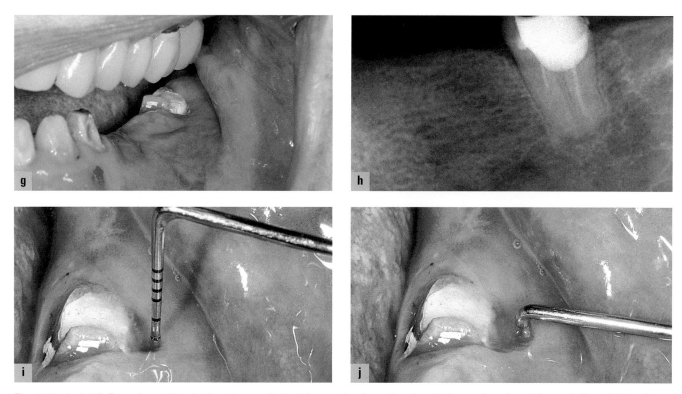

Figs 4-11g to 4-11j Excessive probing depth at the mandibular left second molar and copious drainage of pus from this area indicated this molar as the source of the swelling. Irrigation and drainage resulted in swift reduction of swelling in the entire area along with considerable and immediate relief for the patient. This was diagnosed as a lesion of endodontic origin that had spread anteriorly and found drainage points far removed from its source. Extraction of the molar resolved the symptoms.

Figs 4-12a to 4-12e *(a to c)* Probing pattern typical of an endo-perio case. *(d)* While probing depth is minimal elsewhere, the probe sinks deeply at a single area of the maxillary left canine. *(e)* A radiograph shows an extensive area of radiolucency extending apicomarginally from the endodontically treated canine, which serves as an abutment for the distal extension of an FPD. The pattern of probing plus the considerable extrusion of sealant from the apex, indicating questionable previous RCT, all concurred to limit the diagnosis to either periodontal lesion of endodontic origin or vertical root fracture.

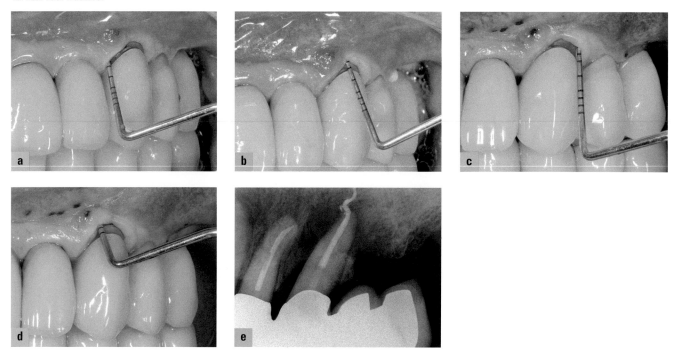

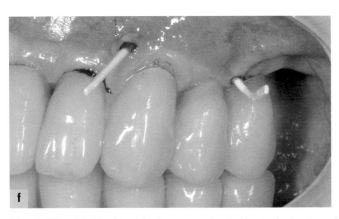 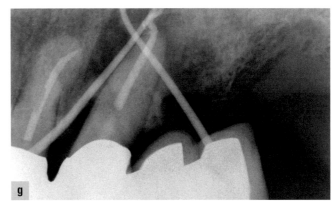

Figs 4-12f and 4-12g Multiple sinus tracts. In addition to the two traced with gutta-percha points, another was observed draining into the sulcus of the maxillary left canine (see Fig 4-12d).

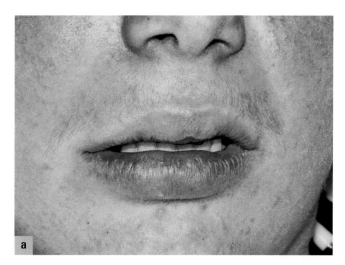

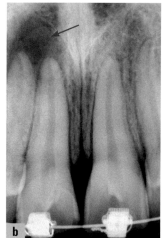

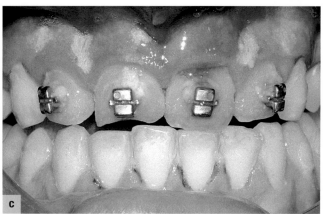

Figs 4-13a to 4-13c *(a)* Young patient with swelling of upper lip. *(b)* Radiograph shows a radiolucency *(red arrow)* at the apices of the maxillary right incisors. *(c)* With the archwire removed, examination reveals inflammation and exudate *(white arrow)* at the gingival margin of the left central incisor. The right central incisor shows signs of previous trauma and did not respond to EPT. The left central incisor responded normally to vitality testing. An unusual case of an acute apical lesion from the necrotic right central incisor draining into the sulcus of the vital left central incisor. (Courtesy of Dr Piero Alessandro Marcoli.)

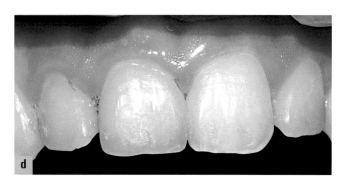

Figs 4-13d to 4-13g Radiographs show gradual disappearance of the apical lesion 6 months, 1 year, and 4 years, respectively, after RCT of the maxillary right central incisor. *(g)* Intraoral examination 4 years posttreatment indicates a return to healthy gingival structure despite poor overall oral hygiene.

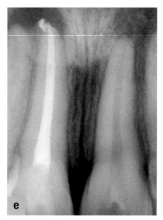

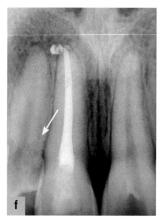

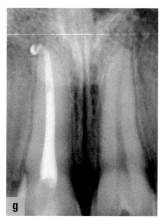

Class 1: Crown-Down Plaque-Induced Periodontal Lesions

The term *crown-down* is borrowed from the endodontic lexicon but in this case describes a periodontal lesion that arises at the gingival margin and progresses apically. It is characterized by colonization of bacterial plaque and calculus on root surfaces, destruction of the attachment apparatus, and consequent apical migration of the junctional epithelium. As the lesion progresses apically, advancing involvement of periradicular tissue may cause it to be mistaken for a Class 2 down-crown lesion (Fig 4-14).

Diagnostic criteria

Findings on probing
Pockets tend to have a broad configuration, narrowing towards the apex. The symptomatic tooth may be part of an overall picture of poor periodontal health.

Endodontic evaluation
Pulpal vitality tests on Class 1 lesions should be normal. If so, the tooth can be said to exhibit a pseudo endo-perio profile with a final diagnosis of crown-down pathology (see Fig 5-1). Further investigation is warranted if there is the slightest suspicion of underlying endodontic involvement upon vitality testing, which would rule out a Class 1 crown-down lesion in favor of a Class 3 combined endo-perio lesion.

Fig 4-14 Class 1 crown-down plaque-induced periodontal lesion.

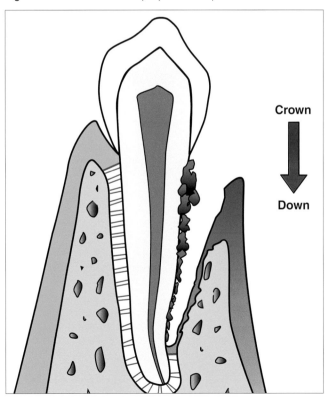

Class 2: Down-Crown Periodontal Lesions of Endodontic Origin

Because the destruction caused by a periodontal lesion of endodontic origin begins apically and advances coronally, these lesions will be labeled *down-crown*. When the damage extends past the periodontium into the surrounding alveolar bone, it develops centrifugally, enlarging outward from its point of origin (Fig 4-15). However, in the current context, discussion will be limited to development of lesions from the apex towards the coronal region, hence the term *down-crown* (Fig 4-16).

Lesions classified as down-crown originate within a closed space, the pulp cavity. They also spread within the limited capacity of the PDL space before entering the surrounding alveolar bone. Down-crown lesions are histologically capable of causing periodontal tissue inflammation but will not lead to irreversible loss of attachment unless left untreated.[58]

Diagnostic criteria

Endodontic evaluation

Inclusion in Class 2 is based on an assumption of pulp necrosis. The pulp will not respond to the electric pulp tester (EPT) or to thermal testing. If the pulp is found to be normal or is determined to have irreversible pulpitis, its inclusion in Class 2 is ruled out.

Pulp testing should be performed when the patient is symptomatic, radiographs show an apical radiolucency or widened PDL space, or in the presence of:

- Previous root canal treatment (RCT) (see Fig 5-19)
- Deep restorations
- Periodontal disease which has advanced to the root apex (see Figs 5-11 and 5-17)
- Ill-fitting crowns or those with deep margins or recurrent decay (see Fig 5-13)

Findings on probing

As discussed above, diagnostic probing in Class 2 situations is in fact instrumentation of a sinus tract (Fig 4-17) rather than probing of a periodontal pocket associated with attachment apparatus loss. A Class 2 lesion is typified by uniform probing depths except for the point at which the probe sinks into the draining tract (Fig 4-18).

Pus drainage from the sinus tract is a sign of acute infection; the infection may subside either spontaneously or with antibiotic treatment. Once the acute stage is past, the sinus tract may shrink or disappear, causing difficulty in locating its opening into the mucosa or gingival sulcus. If a sinus tract is known to be present but sealed off by the crevicular epithelium, it must be reopened with a probe to gain access.

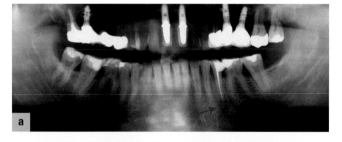

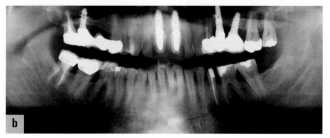

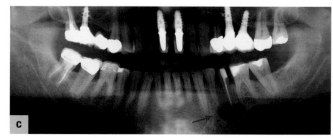

Fig 4-15 *(a to c)* Chronologic panoramic radiographs depicting a lesion of endodontic origin at the apex of the mandibular left second premolar, enlarging outward from its point of origin.

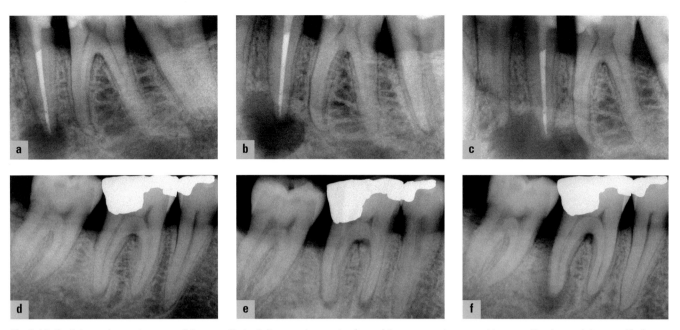

Fig 4-16 Radiolucencies at the apex of the mandibular left second premolar *(a to c)* do not extend to crestal bone, unlike those of the mandibular right first molar *(d to f)* in which the radiolucency spreads coronally. The need for differential diagnosis is greater in such cases.

Fig 4-17 Sagittal *(a)* and frontal *(b)* views illustrating tube-like probing in a typical Class 2 down-crown periodontal lesion of endodontic origin.

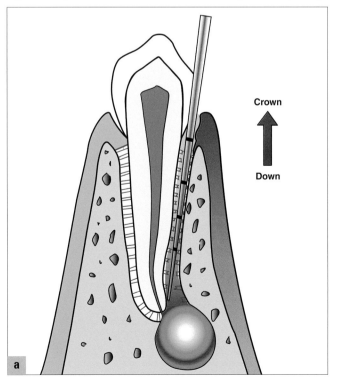

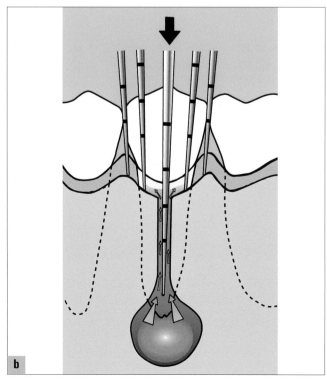

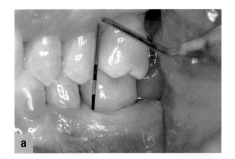 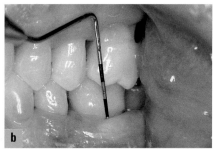 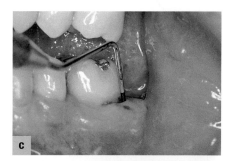

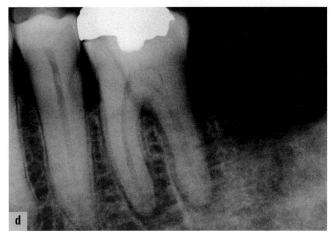 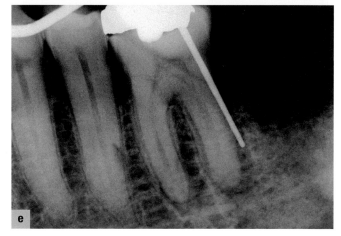

Fig 4-18 In an overall healthy periodontium *(a and b)*, there is a single area where the probe sinks deeply into a narrow orifice *(c)*. *(d and e)* The probe follows the path of a sinus tract towards the apex.

Class 3: Combined Endo-Perio Lesions

When pulpal and periodontal diseases occur concurrently, the diagnostic picture may be unclear. Periodontal probing reveals apparent loss of attachment, often significant; the results of pulp vitality testing may be ambiguous. Arriving at a perfect understanding of the etiopathogenesis may be difficult (Fig 4-19).

Idealized Class 3 profile

A strict interpretation of Class 3 requires detection of both plaque-induced and endodontic pathology within the context of a single periodontal lesion. Criteria for diagnosis are:

• Apical or periradicular lesion compatible with encroaching pulp necrosis
• Loss of attachment
• Periodontal pockets that begin broadly before evenly and gradually narrowing towards the apex, where the probe sinks into a narrow orifice (Fig 4-20) leading to the apical lesion

Clinically common Class 3 profiles

In an ideal picture of pathology, symptoms and clinical findings lead directly to an indisputable diagnosis. In reality, the diagnostic results indicating a possible Class 3 combined endo-perio lesion will be ambiguous. Following are two theoretical case presentations: endodontic diagnosis is the priority in the first, and periodontal diagnosis takes precedence in the second.

Primary concern: Endodontic evaluation

In a hypothetical clinical situation, the patient presents with pain associated with a crowned mandibular molar. Radiographs reveal a distinct radiolucency extending from the apex to crestal bone. The tooth is not responsive to thermal testing or EPT. A cavity test is performed in which a small hole is cut, without anesthetic, through the crown to dentin. Stimulation of dentin will provoke a painful response in a vital tooth. If the tooth in question responds to the cavity test, the pulp diagnosis is normal and treatment of a Class 1 crown-down lesion should be initiated.

If there is no response to the cavity test, pulp necrosis is diagnosed. Although unrelated periodontal disease may be manifest at the same tooth, endodontic treatment should be initiated first[9] followed by a period of waiting.[59]

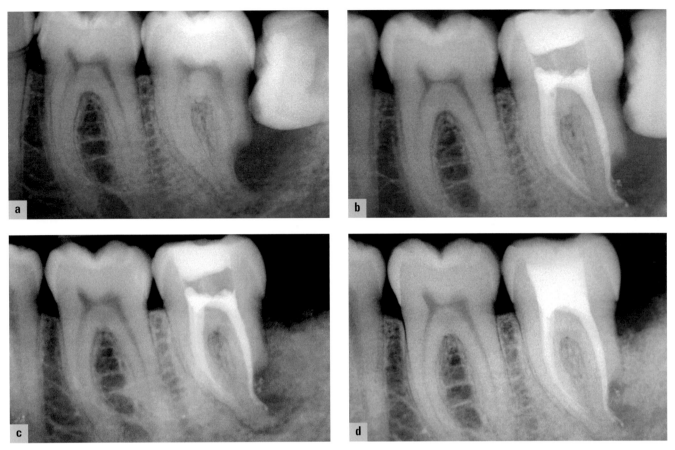

Figs 4-19 *(a)* Extensive endo-perio lesion of the mandibular left second molar with distal pocket depth of 12 mm caused by impaction of the adjacent third molar. *(b)* Completed endodontic treatment of the second molar. Treatment of the distal canal was difficult due to major root resorption. *(c)* Extraction of the third molar and grafting with autologous bone and Bio-Oss (Osteohealth) in a 1:1 ratio. *(d)* Follow-up after 16 months. (Courtesy of Dr M. Badino.)

Fig 4-20 Sagittal *(a)* and frontal *(b)* views illustrating an idealized Class 3 combined endo-perio lesion. At the bottom of the existing plaque-induced pocket, the probe sinks deeply into the narrow orifice of a sinus tract draining a lesion of endodontic origin.

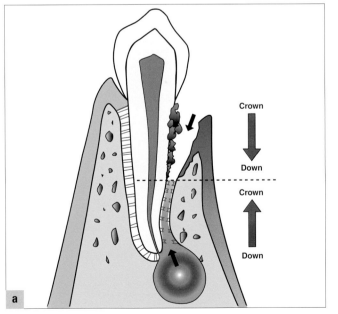

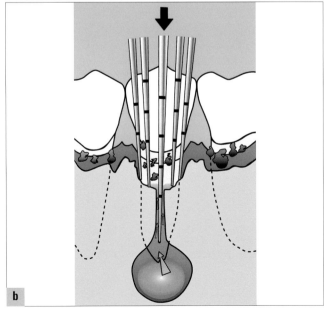

The periodontal situation is reevaluated and treated as necessary. If periodontal resolution follows successful endodontic therapy, then the after-the-fact diagnosis is Class 2 down-crown pathology.

If the results of pulp testing are ambiguous, the tooth is much more likely to belong in the Class 3 category. Hypothetically, in a molar, a multirooted tooth, one or more canals may be necrotic while other areas of pulp remain vital.[60,61] Pathogens from the periodontal pocket may cause retrograde infection of the pulp through the apex or lateral canals.[9,62] Pulp necrosis tends to spread within the pulp cavity in a crown-down pattern, and the same holds true for necrosis that begins at an infected lateral canal. It follows that pulp tissue in areas coronal to the necrotic point of origin may temporarily remain unaffected, hence the mixed results of EPT and thermal tests.

Although much debated, the Class 3 profile in this case corresponds to primary periodontal disease with secondary endodontic involvement.[9,27,51–53,62–67] From a clinical rather than an academic standpoint, relevant concerns are: *(1)* If the periodontal lesion has not spread beyond the root apex and if the tooth responds in any way to vitality testing, it should be treated as a live tooth unless proven otherwise; *(2)* If the lesion has affected the apex, and guided tissue regeneration to regain improved attachment levels is planned, preliminary root canal treatment should be performed in accordance with the golden rule "endo first, then perio"[9] because it is impossible to verify the true vitality of the entire coronal and radicular pulp, especially in multirooted teeth.[60,61]

Primary concern: Findings upon probing

In a second hypothetical situation, a patient presents with a tooth that, upon initial probing, has a pocket consistent with chronic plaque-induced periodontal disease. Upon more careful examination, the apical portion of the pocket leads to another opening which is narrower than the first and whose sides are more parallel. This finding is not entirely compatible with the tube-like pocket associated with the sinus tract of a lesion of endodontic origin. It is therefore necessary to proceed with identification of this phenomenon according to three possible circumstances.

Unusual Presentation

Option one

The lesion is not Class 3 combined endo-perio, as suspected upon probing, but merely an unusual presentation of a Class 1 crown-down lesion (Fig 4-21a). Whether for reasons of plaque and calculus accumulation, of resistance on the part of the attachment apparatus, or of root morphology, the pocket has not developed the expected structure and configuration (see Fig 4-14).

Option two

The periodontal lesion under investigation is the dual result of a plaque-induced periodontal pocket coronally and a lesion of endodontic origin apically, with a sinus tract erupting into the base of the already established periodontal pocket (Fig 4-21b). The morphology of the sinus tract may vary according to the infectious process, root anatomy, and resistance of the periodontium. The apicomarginal pathway created by drainage of an endodontic abscess is facilitated by an attachment apparatus debilitated by periodontal disease (see Fig 5-14). This clinical situation corresponds closely to the idealized Class 3 lesion described earlier.

Option three

Plaque accumulation at the gingival margin of a sinus tract secondary to untreated endodontic pathology can allow bacteria to colonize along the root surface, superimposing a periodontal pocket along the tract (Fig 4-22) via attachment loss and apical migration of the junctional epithelium.[6] This clinical situation was described in the chapter 3 discussion of primary endodontic disease with secondary periodontal involvement but is reclassified here as Class 3 combined endo-perio.

In clinical practice, evidence indicates that, in the event of recent sinus tract appearance and effective root canal treatment, permanent damage to the periodontium due to superimposed periodontal involvement is highly unlikely. It has been proposed that the apicomarginal flow of pus from an endodontic abscess prevents the encroachment of bacterial plaque in the opposite direction.[68]

Further theoretical and academic debate will shed no additional light on the subject of endo-perio lesions. The second half of this book presents a sequence of clinical case studies, including the rationale behind the classification of each. ■

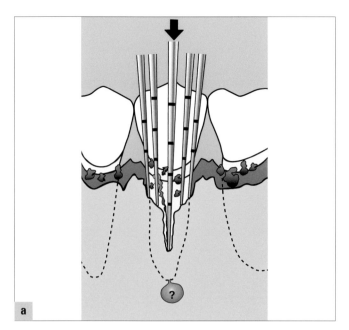 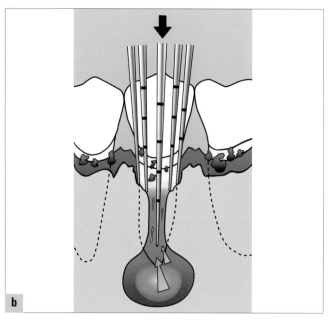

Fig 4-21 *(a)* An unusual presentation of a Class 1 crown-down lesion. A single, narrow area of greater probing depth may appear similar to a sinus tract but instead be secondary to a crack, fracture or abnormally developed groove. *(b)* An unusual presentation of Class 3, combined endo-perio lesion. A particularly aggressive apical abscess may create a wider sinus tract with more divergent walls.

Fig 4-22 An unusual presentation of Class 3, combined endo-perio lesion.

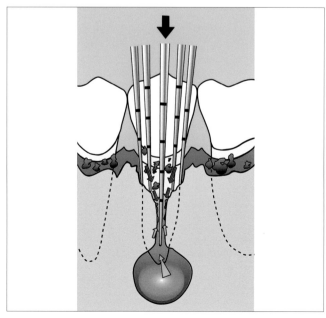

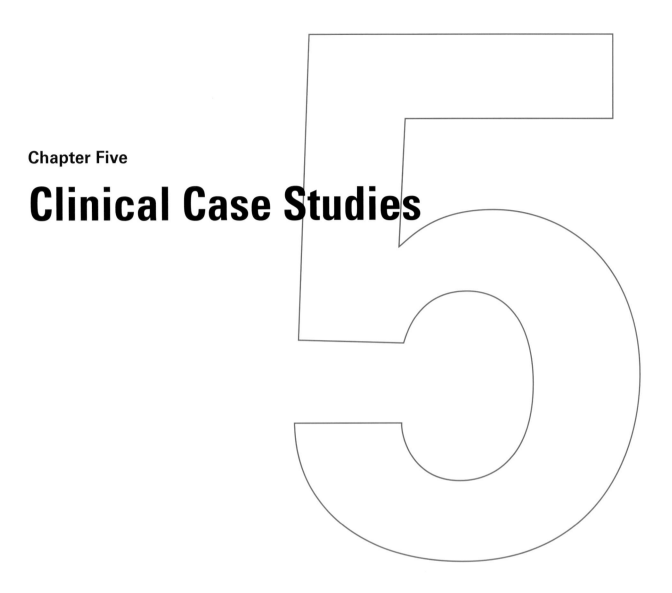

Chapter Five

Clinical Case Studies

The term *endo-perio* encompasses a spectrum of oral pathologies and, first and foremost, requires differential diagnostic investigation into the etiopathogenesis of the lesion in question.

Procedure

Preliminary diagnosis

The first two essential diagnostic findings, *(1)* healthy or unhealthy periodontal tissues and *(2)* pulp tissue vitality or necrosis, lead to a pseudo endo-perio diagnosis. Differential diagnosis cannot be suspended at this point; the practitioner must proceed towards division into endo-perio classes, even if the final diagnosis remains pseudo endo-perio:

- Class 1: Crown-down plaque-induced periodontal lesion
- Class 2: Down-crown periodontal lesion of endodontic origin

In Class 1 lesions, the difference between classification into the endo-perio category as opposed to pseudo endo-perio depends on the ease and immediacy with which pulp vitality is ascertained.

At this preliminary diagnosis stage, a tooth with a healthy crown in which pulp necrosis is not suspected and that responds normally to noninvasive pulp vitality testing using a thermal or electric pulp tester (EPT), is defined as a *Class 1 pseudo endo-perio* case.

Conversely, if the tooth shows signs of pulp pathology such as draining sinus tracts, unsuccessful endodontic treatment, or extensive restorations while also not responding to noninvasive pulp vitality testing (ie, presenting a potential lesion of endodontic nature) the *Class 1 endo-perio* profile will be the preliminary diagnosis.

Similarly, when a tooth presents with changes in the periodontium extending apicomarginally but probing is not compatible with chronic periodontal disease, the *Class 2 pseudo endo-perio* hypothesis is applied (see Fig 5-2). If probing depth indicates lesion of attachment, the diagnosis will be *Class 2 endo-perio*.

Although of academic and didactic interest, the distinction between pseudo endo-perio and genuine endo-perio profiles is of little relevance in clinical and practical applications.

Final diagnosis

The final diagnosis, the moment in which the etiopathogenesis of the lesion has been diagnosed with certainty, may not be determined until some or all treatment has been completed.

Pseudo Endo-Perio Lesion Profiles: Case Studies 1 to 6

Clinical case study 1

Clinical and radiologic examination
The mandibular right first molar is slightly mobile; radiographs show a periodontal bony defect along the mesial root. Calculus is detectible on the root surface.

Initial diagnosis: Endo-perio profile

Further investigation is required to ascertain the status of the periodontium and pulp.

Periodontal examination
Figs 5-1a and 5-1b Probing depth along the mesial root is 10 mm; subgingival calculus is present.
Figs 5-1c to 5-1f Generalized periodontal condition is very poor with widespread inflammation and supra- and subgingival calculus. Full mouth plaque score (FMPS) and full mouth bleeding score (FMBS) greater than 50%. Gingival recession and significant probing depths recorded in a number of sites.

Preliminary treatment choice
Treatment to include management of periodontal disease with scaling and root planing, patient education, and a program of periodontal hygiene maintenance.

Treatment objectives
To eliminate periodontal inflammation and to bring FMPS and FMBS under 20%, reduce probing depths, regain some clinical attachment, and achieve acceptable and continued hygiene maintenance.

Figs 5-1a and 5-1b

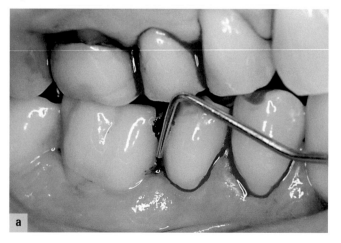

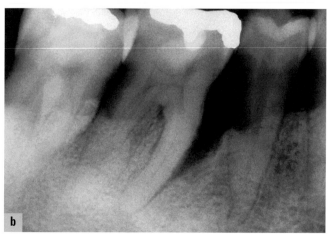

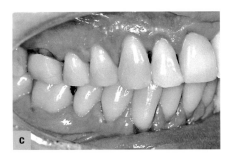
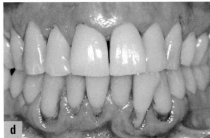
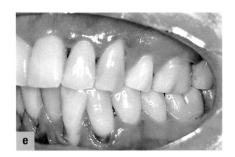

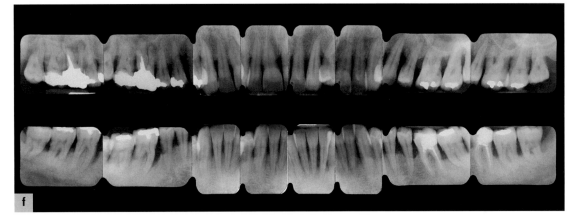

Figs 5-1c to 5-1f

Endodontic examination

The mandibular left first molar responded normally to thermal and EPT testing. In the endo-perio context, immediate confirmation of pulp vitality along with significant probing depths consistent with radiologic evidence resolves any diagnostic doubt.

Preliminary diagnosis: Pseudo endo-perio profile
Final diagnosis: Class 1 plaque-induced periodontal lesion

Figs 5-1g to 5-1l Following treatment the patient was reassessed, with considerable improvement in periodontal health noted. Probing depth around the molar in question was reduced from 10 mm to 7 mm.

Figs 5-1g to 5-1l

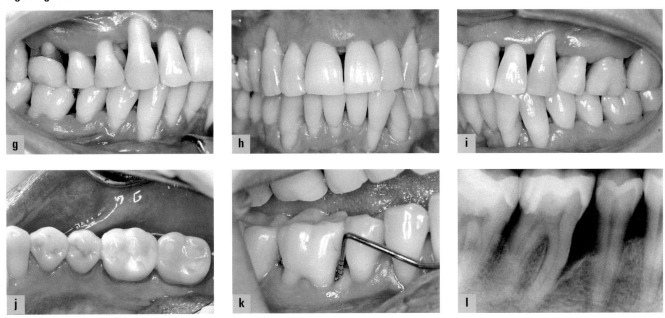

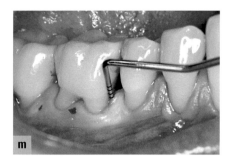 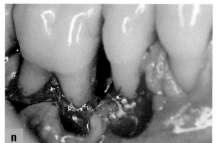 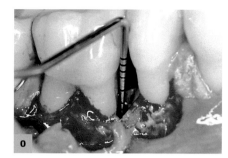

Figs 5-1m to 5-1o

Figs 5-1p to 5-1u

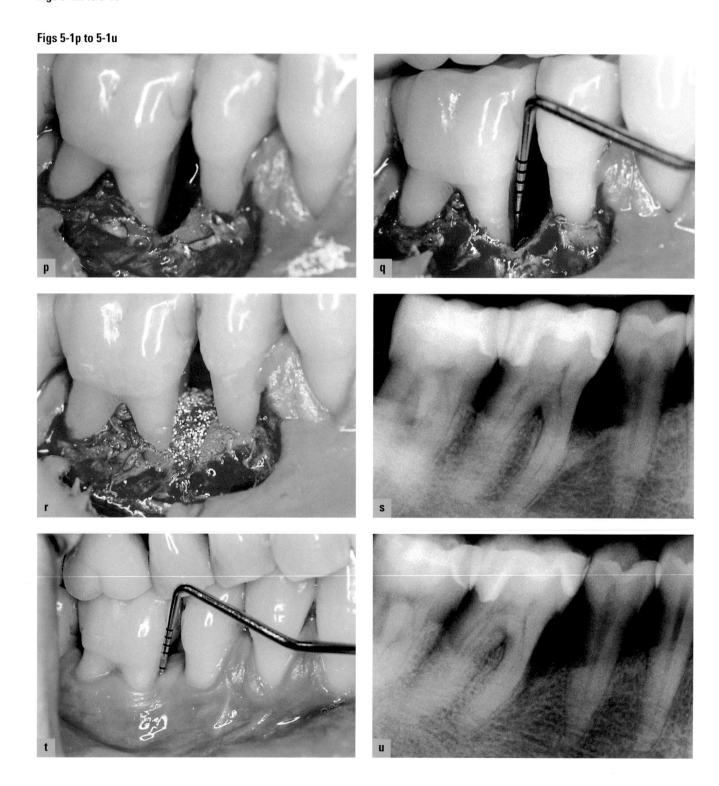

Figs 5-1m to 5-1o Regenerative surgery. Note presence of calculus on the mesial root of the first molar despite repeated scaling and root planing.[69–71]

Figs 5-1p to 5-1u *(p to s)* After thorough scaling and root planing, the osseous defect was filled with autogenous bone and alloplastic material *(t and u)* One-year follow-up shows appreciable reduction in probing depth from 10 mm to 5 mm, along with healthy periodontal tissue free from signs of inflammation.

Figs 5-1v to 5-1y Clinical and radiologic comparison of preoperative *(v and w)* and 1-year postoperative records *(x and y)*.

Figs 5-1v to 5-1y

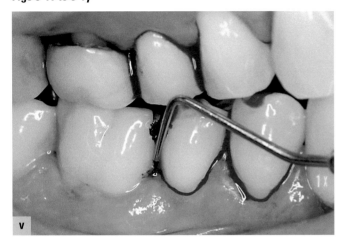

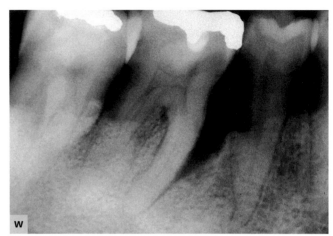

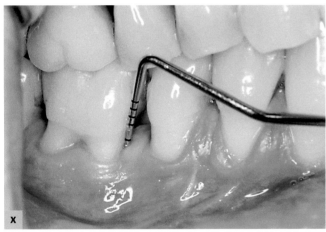

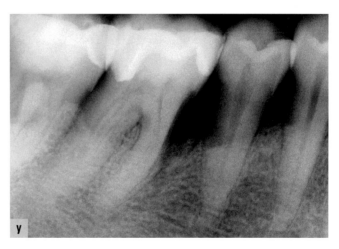

Clinical case study 2

Clinical and radiologic examination
Figs 5-2a and 5-2b The mandibular right third molar is tender to palpation, mobile, and surrounded by acutely inflamed gingiva. Radiographs show an apical radiolucency and widening of the periodontal ligament (PDL) space.

Initial diagnosis: Endo-perio profile

Periodontal examination
Probing depths within normal limits rule out a crown-down plaque-induced lesion. The patient's relatively good overall periodontal condition makes the presence of a single periodontal lesion of such vast proportions highly unlikely.

Endodontic examination
The tooth presented with a sizable amalgam restoration placed 2 years previously. The patient reported that the tooth had been particularly sensitive for some time. There was no

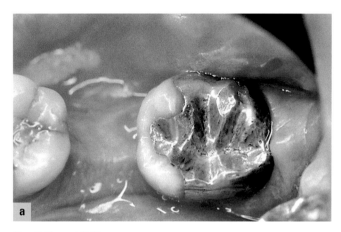
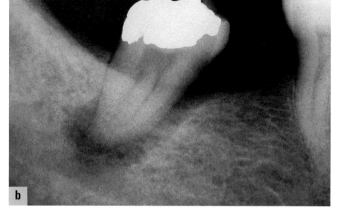

Figs 5-2a and 5-2b

Figs 5-2c to 5-2g

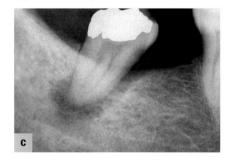
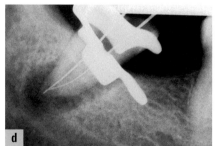
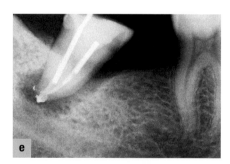

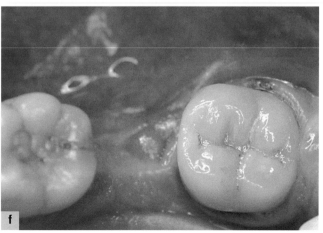
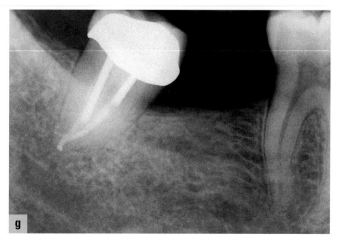

response to thermal testing and EPT. In an endo-perio context, marginal periodontal integrity combined with a high probability of necrotic pulp immediately removed diagnostic doubt. A negative response to invasive pulp cavity testing confirmed pulp necrosis and clarified the diagnosis.

Figs 5-2c to 5-2g *(c to e)* Stages of endodontic treatment. *(f and g)* Two-year follow-up shows complete healing of the periodontium.

Preliminary diagnosis: Pseudo endo-perio profile
Final diagnosis: Class 2 periodontal lesion of endodontic origin in the context of a pseudo endo-perio profile

Clinical case study 3

(Courtesy of Dr Fabio Gorni.)

Figs 5-3a and 5-3b The mandibular left second premolar is the mesial abutment for a three-unit fixed partial denture (FPD). *(a)* Apicomarginal radiolucency. Despite a first impression of pseudo endo-perio profile, the presence of inadequate previous root canal treatment (RCT) and absence of significant probing depths define the lesion's origin as endodontic. *(b)* The successful outcome of proper endodontic treatment confirmed the diagnosis as a Class 2 periodontal lesion of endodontic origin.

Figs 5-3a and 5-3b

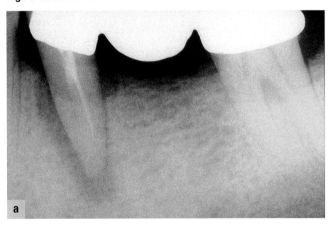

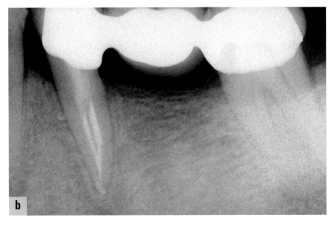

Clinical case study 4

Note: A sinus tract typically leads to a periodontal lesion of endodontic origin with its orifice facial to the affected tooth.
Figs 5-4a and 5-4b A sinus tract draining slightly distal to the maxillary right lateral incisor. Probing depths were within normal limits. The sinus tract led to a periodontal lesion of endodontic origin.
Figs 5-4c to 5-4g (*c to e*) Stages of apicoectomy and postoperative radiograph. *(f and g)* Three-year follow-up shows healing of the endodontic lesion despite poorly maintained dental hygiene.

Figs 5-4a and 5-4b

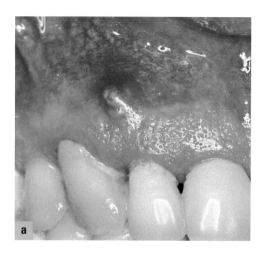 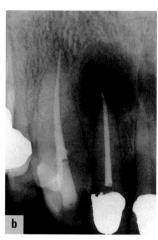

Figs 5-4c to 5-4g

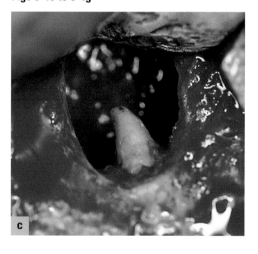 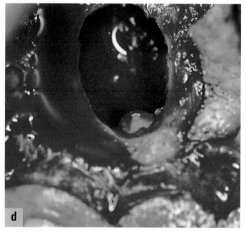 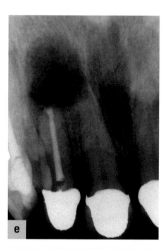

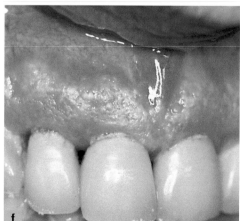 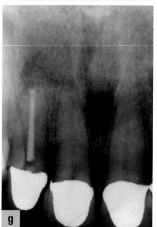

Clinical case study 5

Figs 5-5a to 5-5h *(a)* A 12-year-old female presented with swelling and a sinus tract labial to her maxillary right central incisor. *(b)* The tooth had earlier RCT, and obturation appeared to be inadequate. *(c and d)* Upon access of the pulp cavity, a considerable quantity of pus discharged. *(e to h)* The previously placed filling material, presumably Thermafil (Dentsply), was removed, and the canal reinstrumented and sealed with thermoplastic gutta-percha. Follow-up one week later showed resolution of the labial gingival swelling and disappearance of the sinus tract.

Figs 5-5a to 5-5h

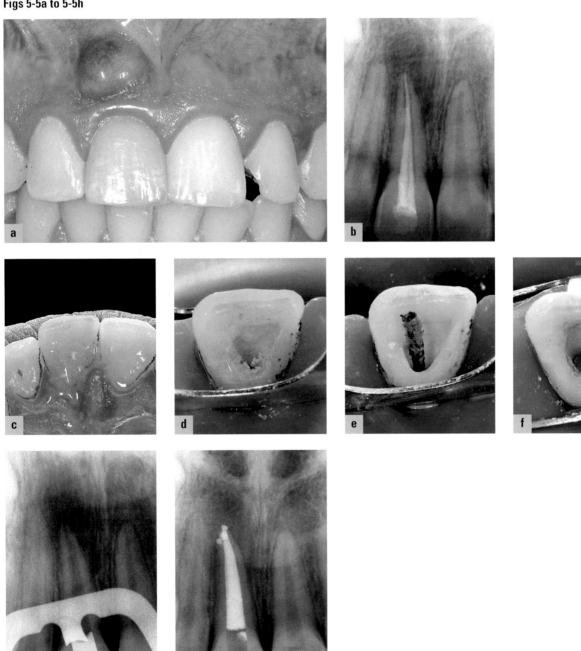

Figs 5-5i to 5-5l (*i and j*) Conservative restoration of the lingual access preparation. *(k and l)* Three months posttreatment.

Figs 5-5i to 5-5l

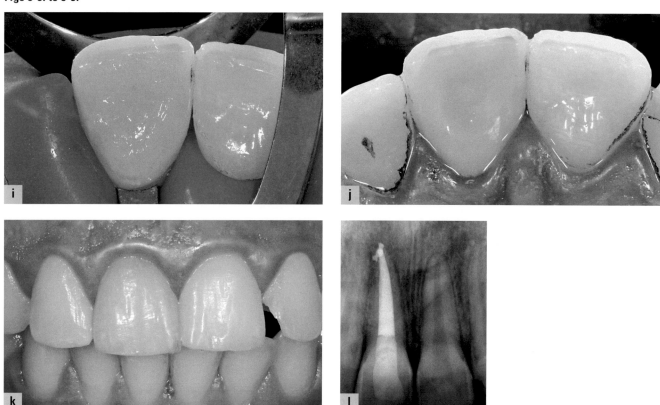

Clinical case study 6

Figs 5-6a to 5-6d (*a and d*) Pseudo endo-perio lesion of the mandibular left incisors with draining sinus tract. In some cases an abscess will form in a plaque-induced periodontal lesion context. (*c and d*) Radiographs show apicomarginal periodontal damage compatible with an endo-perio profile, requiring further investigation into the nature of the lesion.

Figs 5-6a to 5-6d

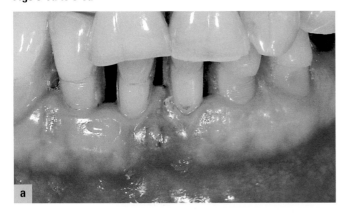
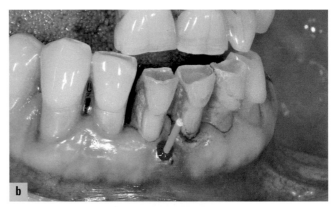
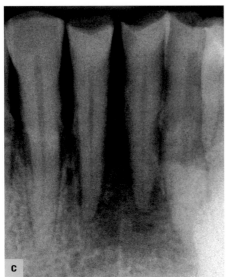
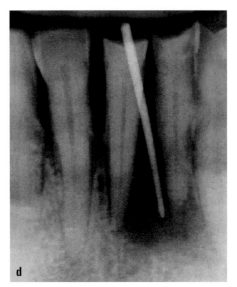

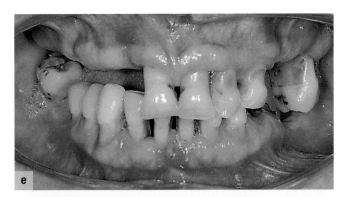

Figs 5-6e to 5-6k Considerations contributing to the diagnosis include generally poor periodontal health with visible and radiologic evidence of calculus on root surfaces *(e and f)*, location of sinus tract *(g and h)*, and findings on probing *(i). (j and k)* Teeth adjacent to the draining sinus had a normal response to invasive cavity testing, confirming the plaque-induced nature of the lesion responsible for the sinus tract.

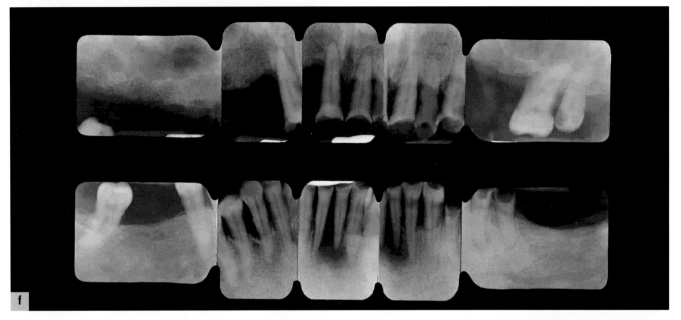

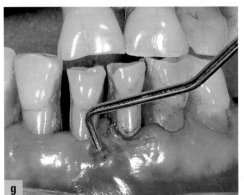

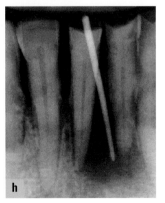

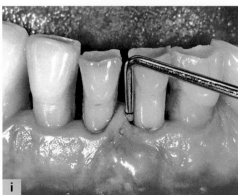

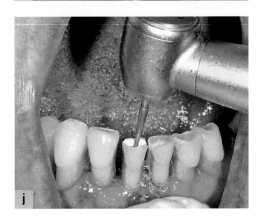

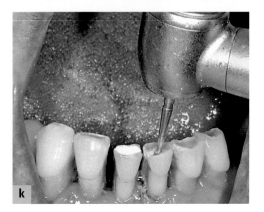

Pseudo Endo-Perio Lesion Profiles: Clinical Case Studies 7 to 9

The formation of a draining sinus tract indicates the presence of an abscess caused by either periodontal or endodontic pathology. The location of its orifice is often indicative of its etiology: the sinus tract from an abscess due to a periodontal lesion of endodontic origin is usually located more apically, while those due to plaque-induced periodontal pathology are generally located closer to the gingival margin.

However, there are situations in which the location of the sinus tract does not help form an accurate diagnosis. From an endo-perio point of view, it should be remembered that a lesion may be centered buccally or lingually and may not be radiologically visible. Consequently, there are certain clinical situations in which sinus tracts draining in unusual locations make a correct diagnosis more difficult.

Clinical case study 7

Figs 5-7a to 5-7f Sinus tract draining paramarginal and mesiobuccal to the maxillary right lateral incisor, an endodontically treated tooth with a radiologically normal apex.

Final diagnosis: Class 1 plaque-induced periodontal lesion in a pseudo endo-perio context

Figs 5-7a to 5-7f

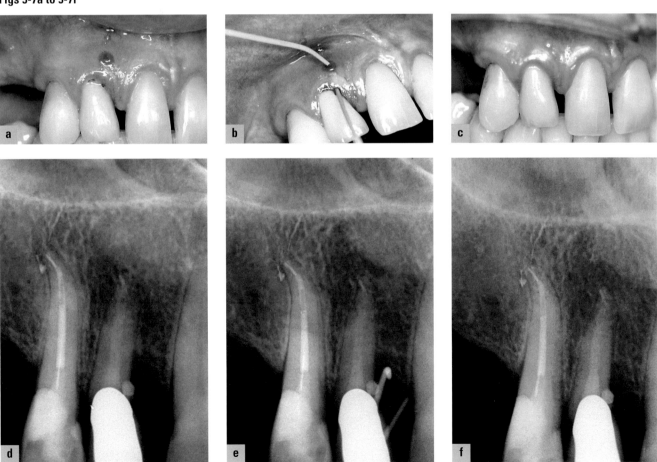

Clinical case study 8

Figs 5-8a and 5-8b (*a*) Lesion runs buccal to a maxillary right central incisor that had been treated with RCT and restored with a carbon-fiber core and metal-ceramic FPD. (*b*) Normal instrumentation and obturation with no periradicular radiolucency. The adjacent left central incisor also had previous RCT, including apicoectomy and retrograde amalgam filling, and a metal-ceramic FPD.

Figs 5-8c to 5-8l (*c to d*) A radiograph taken with a gutta-percha point inserted into the lesion indicated the middle third of the right central incisor as a potential source of the

lesion. (*f and g*) Periodontal probing of both central incisors showed pocket depths no greater than 3 mm. The preliminary diagnosis is Class 2 pseudo endo-perio. (*j to l*) A sulcular incision allowed reflection of an access flap, revealing a soft yellow mass labial to the left central incisor and signs of a lateral canal emerging in the middle third of the right central incisor root. Presence of the lateral canal was confirmed with an endodontic file.

Final diagnosis: Class 2 periodontal lesion of endodontic origin

Figs 5-8a and 5-8b

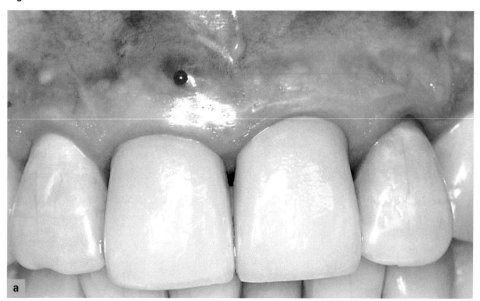
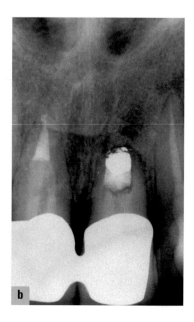

Figs 5-8c to 5-8l

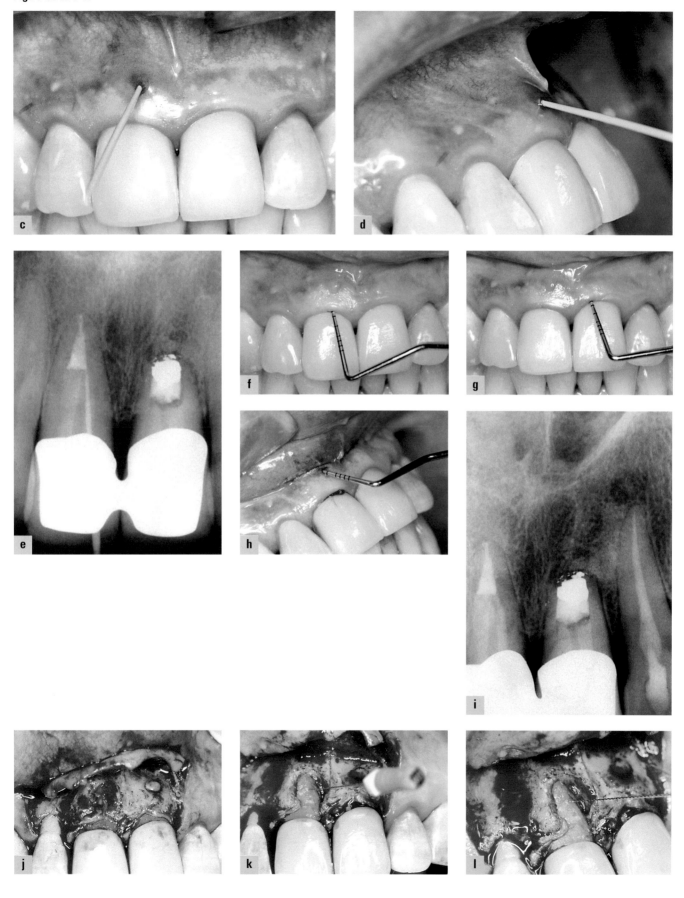

Figs 5-8m to 5-8r *(m to o)* The lateral canal was instrumented with ultrasonic tips and sealed with mineral trioxide aggregate (MTA). *(p and q)* The flap was repositioned and closed with Vicryl sutures (Ethicon). *(r)* Postoperative control radiograph.

Figs 5-8s to 5-8w Follow-up records at 7 months *(s and t)* and 19 months *(u to w)* showed healing and a stable overall condition. The surgical technique avoided unesthetic gingival margin recession. The patient had declined recommended retreatment of the central left incisor; fortunately this tooth appeared asymptomatic during follow-up examination.

Figs 5-8m to 5-8r

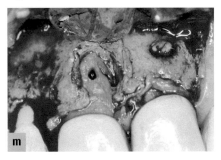

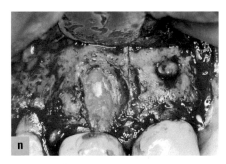

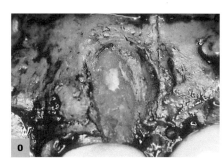

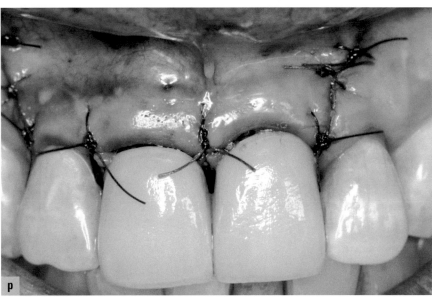

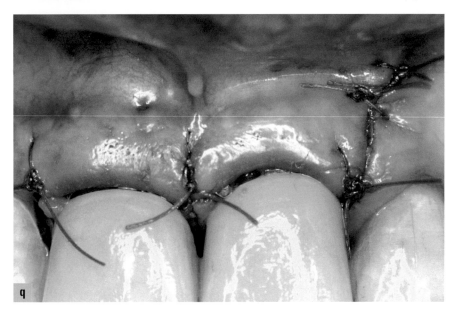

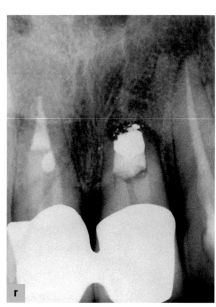

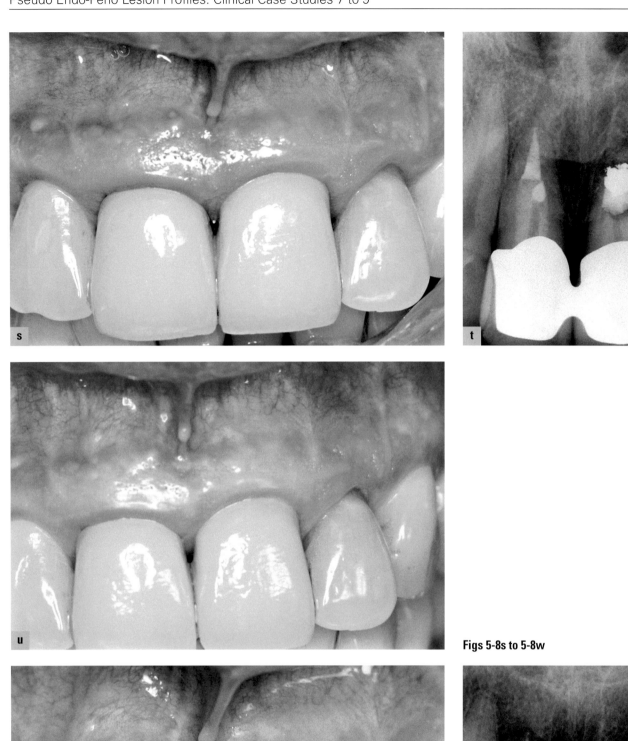

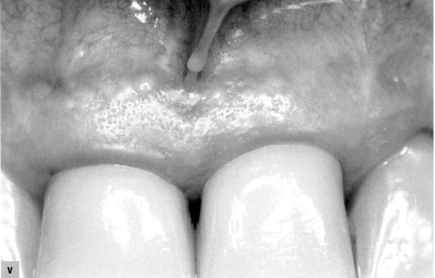

Figs 5-8s to 5-8w

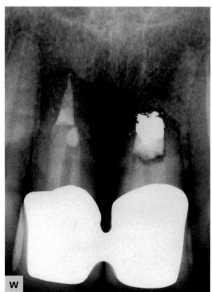

Figs 5-8x to 5-8z At 4 years 5 months posttreatment, the incisors are periodontically and endodontically stable and, in spite of a slight increase in radiolucency distal to the apex of the left incisor, the patient remains free of symptoms.

Figs 5-8x to 5-8z

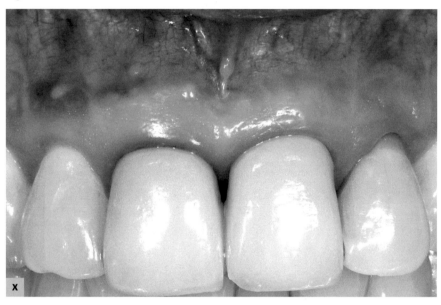

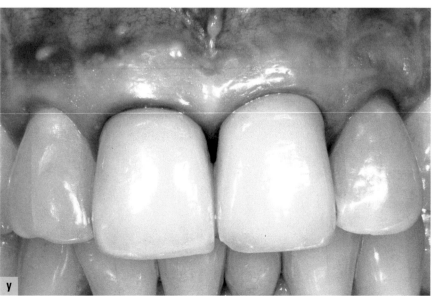

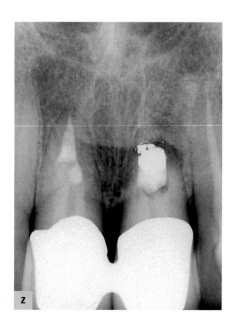

Clinical case study 9

Figs 5-9a to 5-9e Sinus tract draining at a maxillary right central incisor with a conservative distal interproximal composite restoration. *(a and b)* Periodontal probe readings around both central incisors were within normal limits. *(c)* Periradicular radiolucency along the mesial aspect of the right central incisor root and radiolucency in the coronal third of the left central incisor root, which is intact and vital. The patient reported several years of orthodontic treatment completed approximately 10 years earlier. This information suggested that the radiolucency in the left central incisor was compatible with external resorption related to the previous orthodontic work.[16] The patient was warned that the area would require careful monitoring. *(d and e)* A gutta-percha point inserted into the sinus tract corresponded to the suspicious area along the mesial root surface of the right central incisor. This tooth was not responsive to thermal and EPT pulp vitality tests.

Diagnosis: Class 2 periodontal lesion of endodontic origin in a pseudo endo-perio context

Figs 5-9a to 5-9e

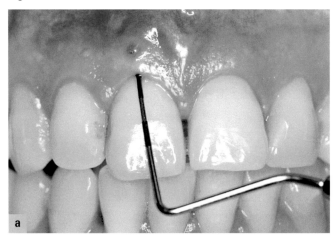

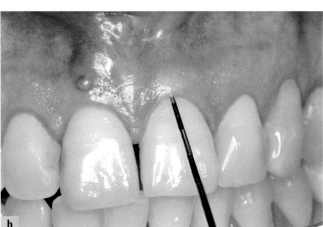

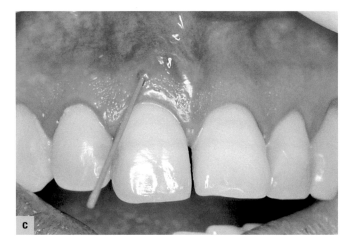

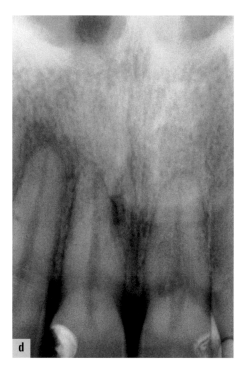

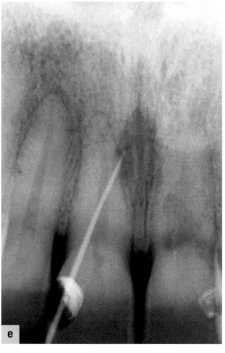

Figs 5-9f to 5-9k *(f to i)* Stages of RCT were followed by conservative restoration with direct composite (Enamel Plus, Micerium). *(j and k)* Radiopaque canal sealant revealed multiple lateral canals presumed to be accountable for the adjacent periradicular lesion.

Figs 5-9f to 5-9k

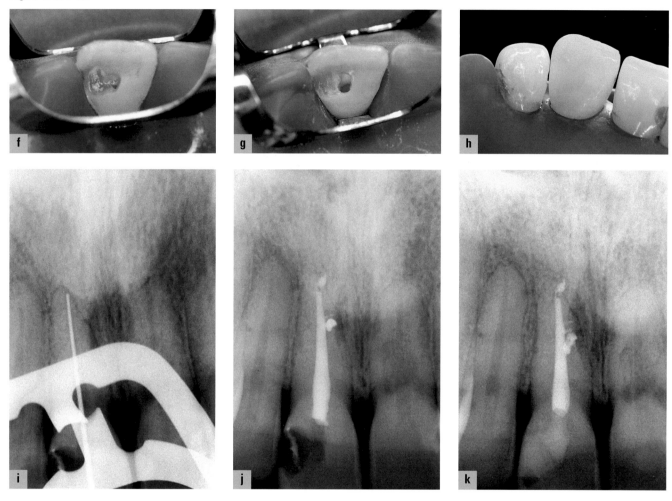

Clinical case study 10: A complex case

Figs 5-10a to 5-10g *(a and b)* Draining sinus tract was found near the maxillary left first premolar *(arrow)*. The tooth had been previously treated with RCT, cast post and core, and metal-ceramic FPD. *(c to g)* This treatment was part of major prosthodontic and periodontal rehabilitation of the maxillary arch extending from the right second premolar to the left second molar.

Figs 5-10a to 5-10g

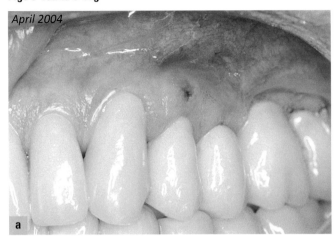

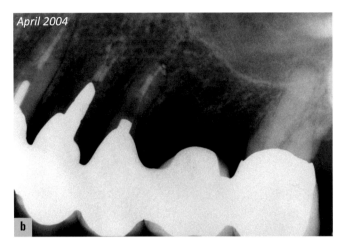

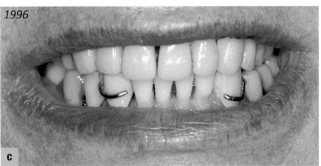

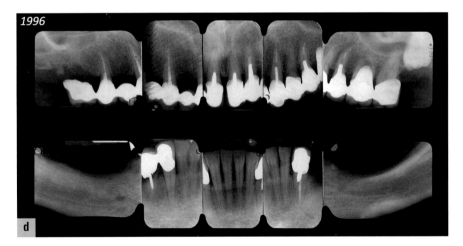

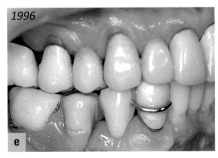

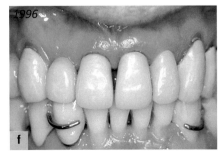

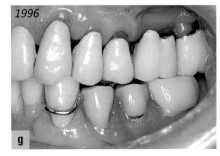

Figs 5-10h to 5-10o Regular follow-ups were without incident
for 8 years *(h to l)*, until the patient presented with the sinus
tract *(m to o; red circle)*.

Figs 5-10h to 5-10o

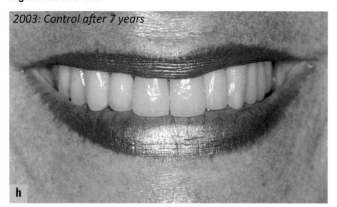

2003: Control after 7 years

h

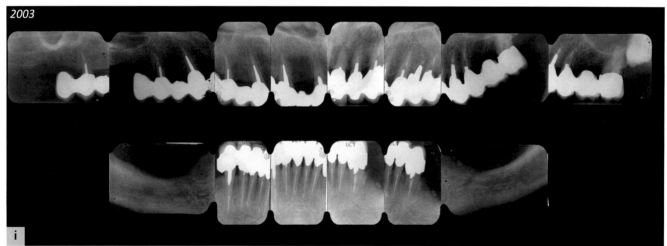

2003

i

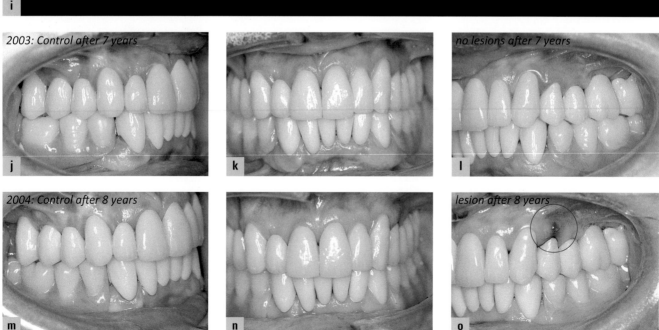

2003: Control after 7 years | | *no lesions after 7 years*

j   k   l

2004: Control after 8 years | | *lesion after 8 years*

m   n   o

Figs 5-10p and 5-10q Both maxillary left premolars had probing depths within normal limits, indicating that neither had a periodontal pocket associated with attachment loss.

Figs 5-10r to 5-10t A gutta-percha point inserted into the lesion corresponded to the middle third of the mesial root surface of the first premolar, adjacent to the apical extent of the post and core.

Preliminary diagnosis: Root fracture as a result of overinstrumentation and/or root perforation

Figs 5-10p and 5-10q

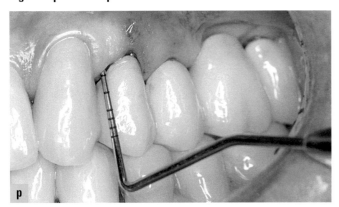

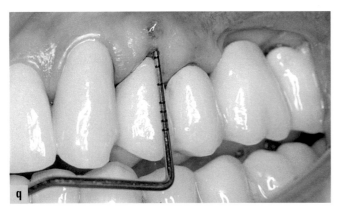

Figs 5-10r to 5-10t

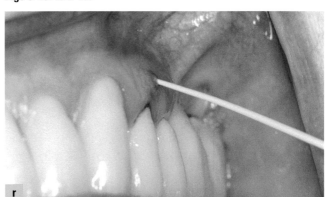

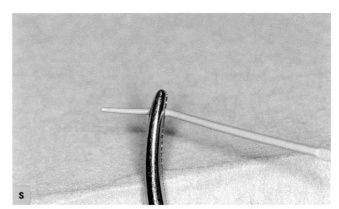

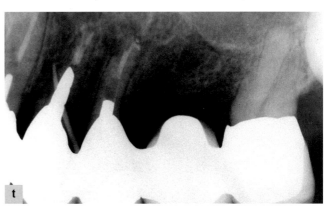

Figs 5-10u to 5-10x Incision and flap reflection revealed root perforation and microfracture near the apical extent of the cast post.

Figs 5-10y to 5-10bb The fracture line was instrumented along its entire length and, at the expense of the cast post

and core, a cavity was created in the root and filled with MTA. While not an accepted use of MTA, no alternatives were available besides extraction. Loss of the first premolar would have required removal of all FPDs in the quadrant, which the patient was not prepared to accept.

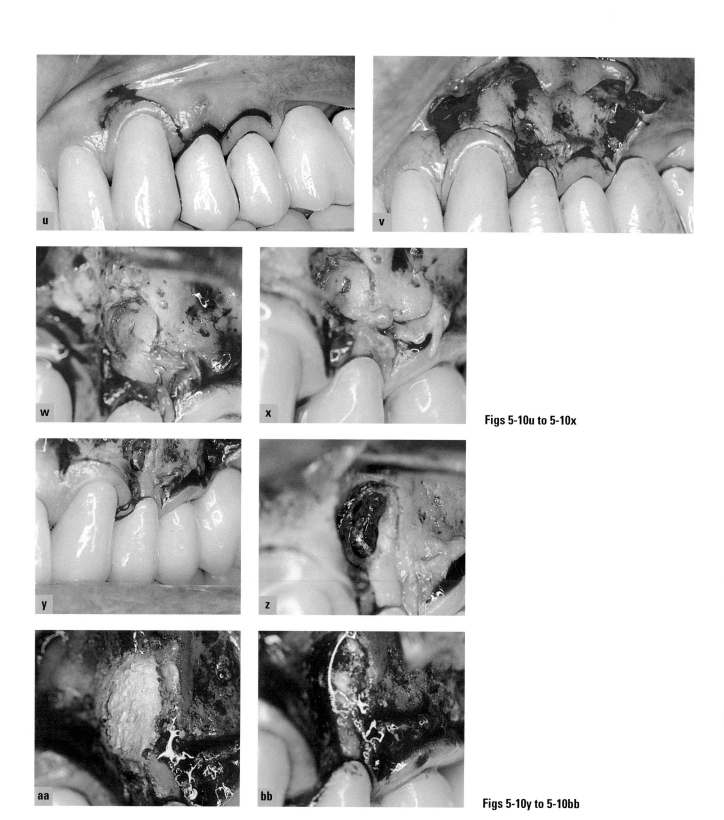

Figs 5-10u to 5-10x

Figs 5-10y to 5-10bb

Figs 5-10cc to 5-10ff The flap was repositioned and closed with 5-0 Vicryl sutures (Ethicon) and is shown immediately *(cc)* and 1 week postoperation *(dd)*. *(ee and ff)* Radiographs taken from two angles confirm MTA placement.

Figs 5-10gg to 5-10jj *(gg)* Two years later, the marginal gingiva of the first premolar is healthy despite the risk of postsurgical recession. *(hh to ii)* The maxillary left second molar, supporting an FPD, was discovered to be carious. *(jj)* The FPD was sectioned distal to the adjacent pontic, and the second molar was extracted.

Figs 5-10cc to 5-10ff

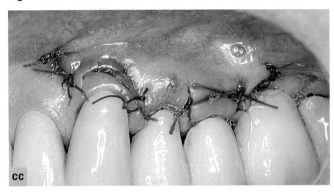

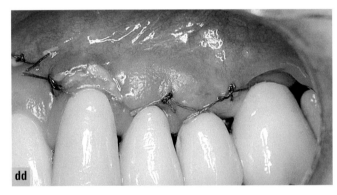

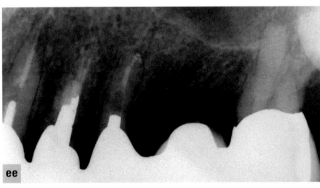

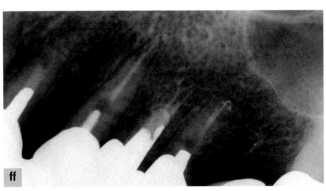

Figs 5-10gg to 5-10jj

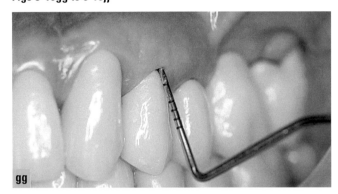

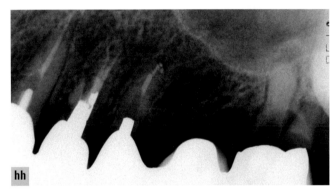

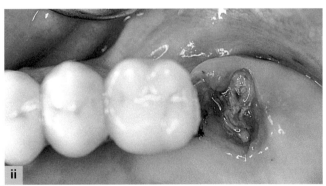

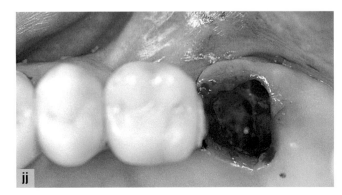

Figs 5-10kk and 5-10ll Two months later, both premolars presented with signs of marginal tissue inflammation and buccal periodontal pockets. Clinical and radiologic evidence strongly suggested root fracture.

Differential diagnosis: Periodontal lesion of endodontic origin vs plaque-induced periodontal lesion vs vertical root fracture

Figs 5-10mm to 5-10pp *(mm to oo)* A flap was reflected, revealing multiple root fractures as suspected. *(pp)* The FPD

was sectioned distal to the maxillary left canine, and the roots of the two premolars were extracted.

Figs 5-10qq to 5-10uu *(qq to ss)* Loss of buccal alveolar bone secondary to the root fracture. *(tt and uu)* The defect was surgically corrected with a ridge-splitting technique that replaced missing buccal bone with palatal alveolar bone.[18]

Figs 5-10vv to 5-10yy *(vv)* Collagen membrane secured with sutures anchored to periosteum. After 2 months, the osseous surgery has recreated an acceptable alveolar crest width despite the original major defect. *(ww to yy)* Further widening of the ridge to prepare for implant placement.

Figs 5-10kk and 5-10ll

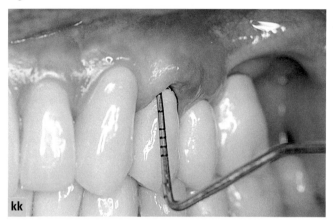
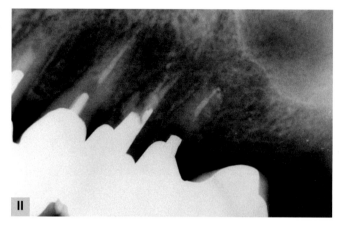

Figs 5-10mm to 5-10pp

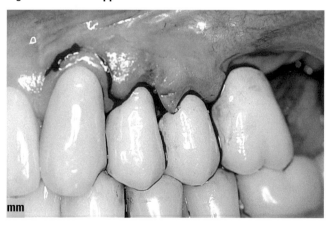
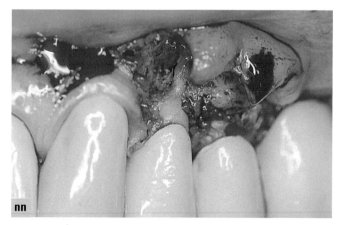

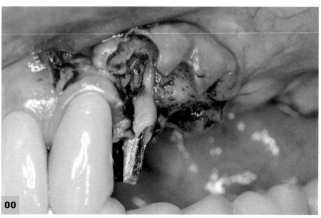
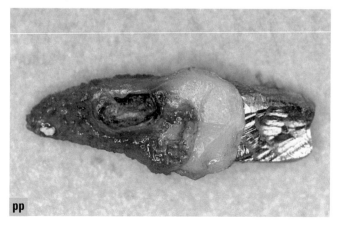

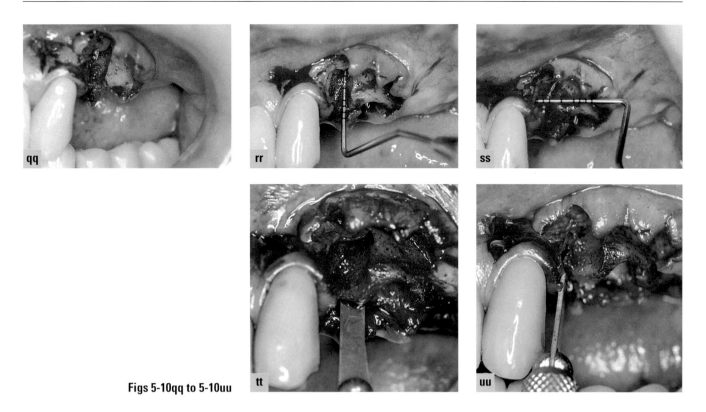

Figs 5-10qq to 5-10uu

Figs 5-10vv to 5-10yy

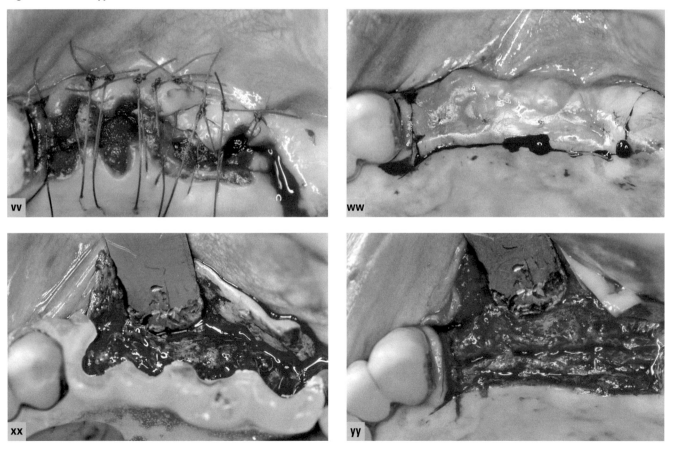

Figs 5-10zz to 5-10ccc Three endosseous implants (Exacta [Biaggini]) were placed. Note how surgery has successfully corrected the osseous defect, rebuilt the natural buccal contours of the ridge, and allowed for placement of implants well aligned for prosthodontic restoration.

Figs 5-10ddd to 5-10ggg Stages of implant restoration. *(ddd)* Final impression stage. Note healthy peri-implant tissue contours and correct positioning of implants. *(eee)* Abutments in place. *(fff and ggg)* Occlusal and facial views of metal-ceramic implant-supported FPD.

Figs 5-10hhh to 5-10kkk Six months posttreatment.

Figs 5-10zz to 5-10ccc

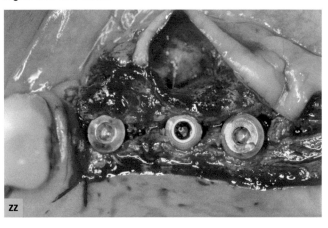

zz

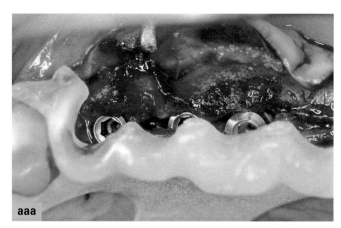

aaa

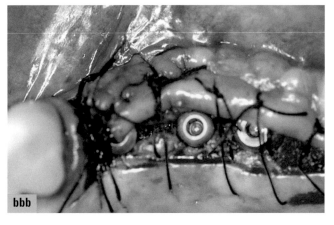

bbb

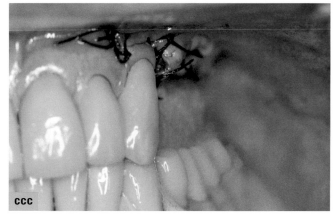

ccc

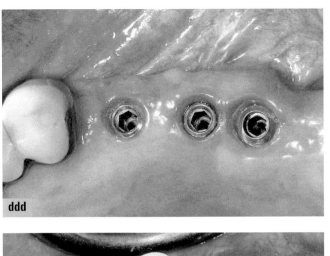

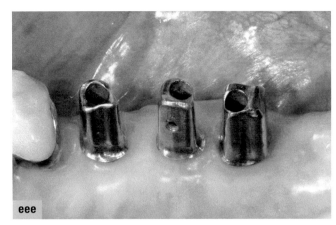

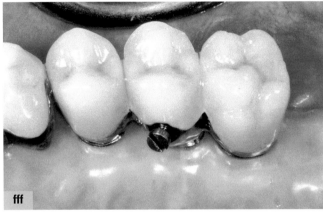

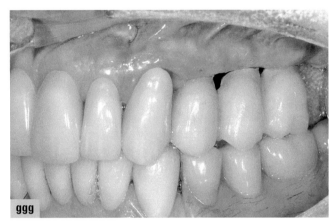

Figs 5-10ddd to 5-10ggg

Figs 5-10hhh to 5-10kkk

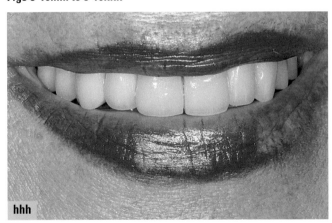

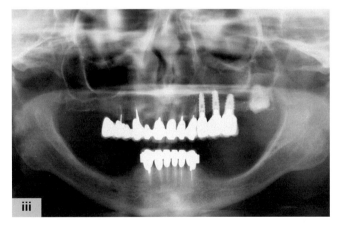

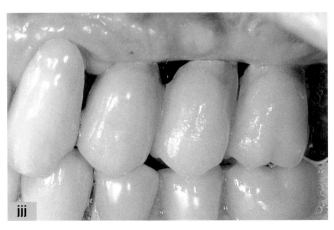

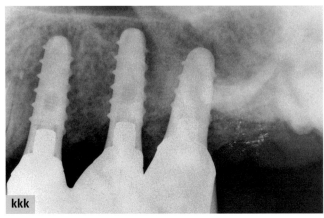

Endo-Perio Lesion Profiles: Clinical Case Studies 11 to 21

Clinical case study 11

Figs 5-11a to 5-11d *(a)* A 51-year-old male patient presented with a deep restoration in his mandibular left third molar. The tooth was very mobile and the surrounding tissues acutely inflamed, with purulent exudate. *(b)* A radiograph showed periapical and periradicular radiolucency and calculus on the mesial root surface, along with evidence of apical root resorption. *(c and d)* Probing revealed significant attachment loss in all areas and caused abundant drainage of pus. The results of noninvasive vitality testing were inconclusive.

Figs 5-11e to 5-11j The patient's overall periodontal health was not good but appeared to be chronic in nature in comparison to the acute condition of the third molar.

Figs 5-11k to 5-11n *(k)* Invasive cavity testing yielded a positive result, indicating a vital pulp. *(l)* The molar was extracted and examined. *(m and n)* The mesial root and its apex showed abundant calculus, likely of a longstanding nature, while the distal root apex was free of visible calculus. Had the mesial root pulp been necrotized and the distal root pulp vital, interpretation of clinical findings could have led to a different diagnosis.

As a purely theoretic exercise, suppose that the pulp had necrotized resulting in a secondary periodontal lesion of endodontic origin within the context of the existing plaque-induced periodontal lesion. From a clinical point of view, this would have been irrelevant, but diagnostically the molar would have been categorized as Class 3 combined endo-perio lesion.

Final diagnosis: Class 1 crown-down periodontal lesion

Figs 5-11a to 5-11d

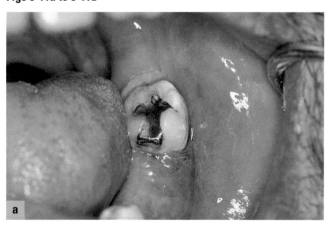

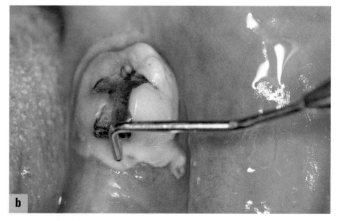

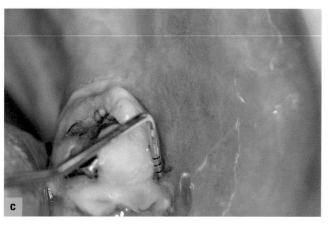

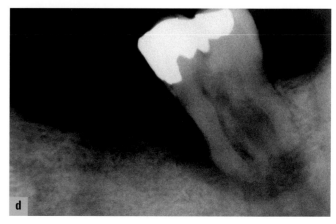

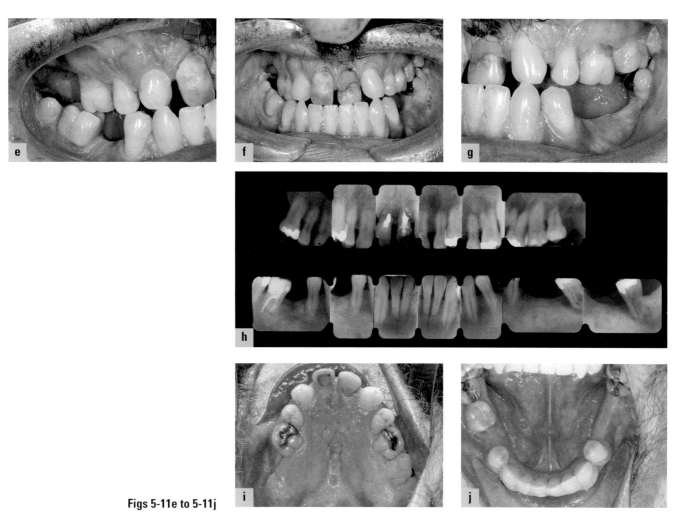

Figs 5-11e to 5-11j

Figs 5-11k to 5-11n

Clinical case study 12

Figs 5-12a and 5-12b *(a)* A 68-year-old male patient presented with inflammation of the tissues surrounding the mandibular left first molar. Frequently, multirooted teeth may have nonvital and vital canals simultaneously. *(b)* Note the generalized periodontal involvement of the distal root, typical of an endo-perio profile. Noninvasive vitality testing was inconclusive but the cavity test was positive, proving pulp vitality.

Figs 5-12c to 5-12g *(c to g)* Whether the positive cavity test response indicated vitality of the entire pulp, or only of a part of it, was immaterial. Treatment entailed RCT of the mesial, periodontally healthy root, plus resection and extraction of the distal root. The mesial root then served as the abutment for an FPD.

Figs 5-12h and 5-12i Four years posttreatment.

Figs 5-12a and 5-12b

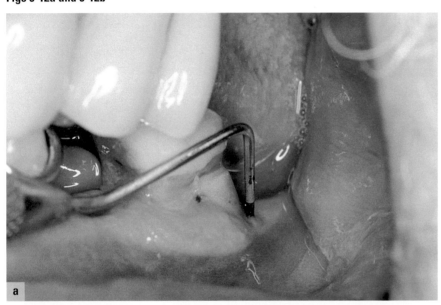

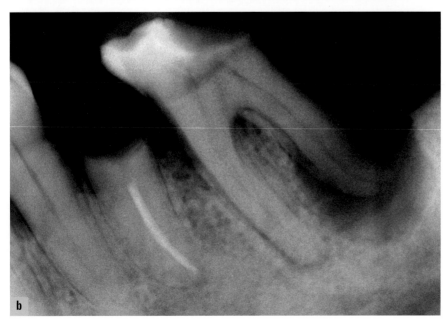

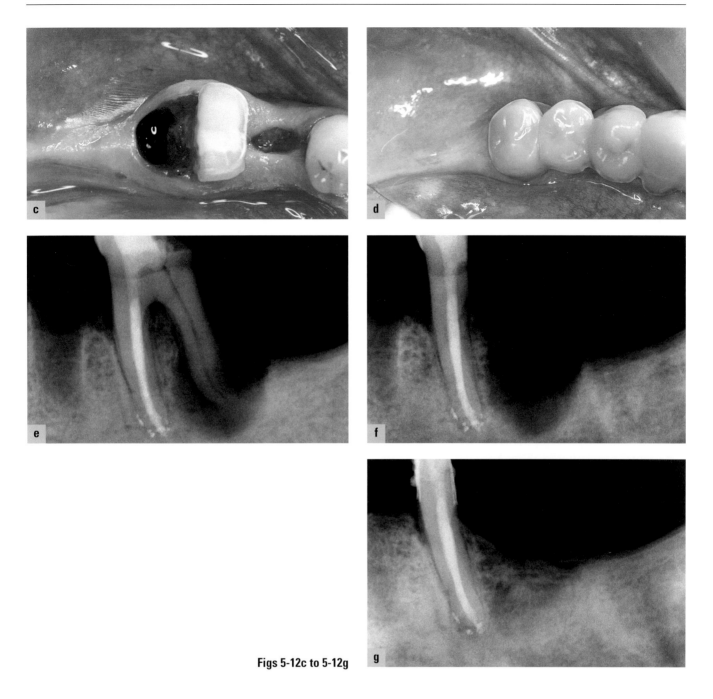

Figs 5-12c to 5-12g

Figs 5-12h and 5-12i

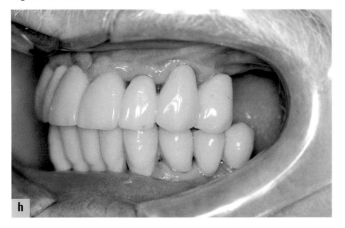

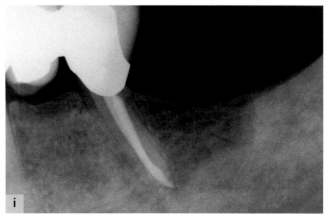

Clinical case study 13

Figs 5-13a to 5-13c *(a and b)* A 72-year-old female patient presented swollen soft tissues surrounding her mandibular left second molar *(white arrows)*, the distal abutment for a metal-ceramic FPD. Although not endodontically treated, the tooth responded negatively to noninvasive vitality testing, an unsurprising result for an extensively restored tooth. A buccal sinus tract led to the furcation. *(c)* Radiologic investigation showed an area of radiolucency *(red arrows)* extending along the coronal half of the mesial root. No apical radiolucency was observed.

Figs 5-13d and 5-13e *(d)* Pocket depths were normal except for the buccal furcation area and at the mesiobuccal line angle, corresponding to the radiolucent area. *(e)* Probing at this point was 9 mm.

Figs 5-13f to 5-13j *(f to h)* Taking into consideration the patient's generally good periodontal health, results of probing, and patient´s history, the decision was made to perform a cavity test. The negative response indicated pulp necrosis and confirmed the diagnosis as a Class 2 downcrown lesion. *(i and j)* Radiographs taken during and after RCT showed that canal sealant had flowed into a large lateral canal *(red arrows)* corresponding to the nearby periodontal lesion.

Figs 5-13k to 5-13n Pretreatment *(k to l)* and posttreatment *(m and n)* documentation demonstrates that the correct diagnosis, therapeutic choice, and properly executed treatment together contribute to reverse the pathology.

Figs 5-13a to 5-13c

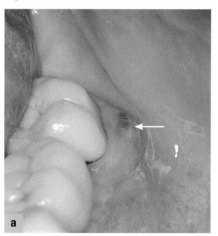
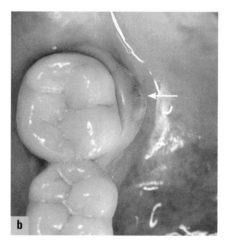
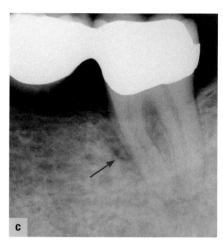

Figs 5-13d and 5-13e

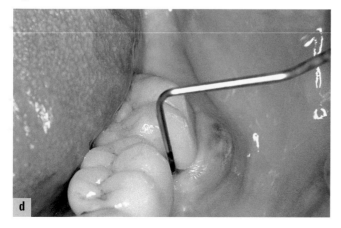
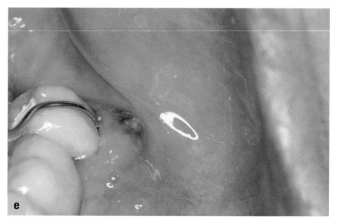

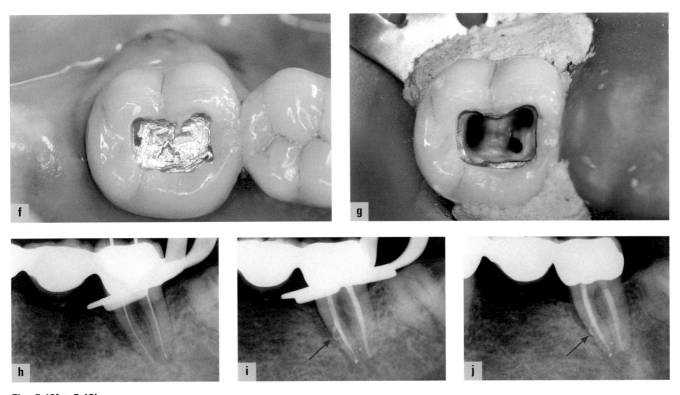

Figs 5-13f to 5-13j

Figs 5-13k to 5-13n

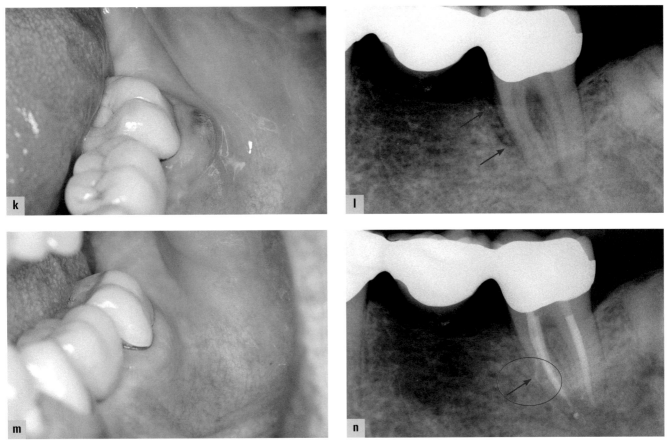

Clinical case study 14

Figs 5-14a to 5-14e Radiographs show the progression of pathology over 6 months in a mandibular right first molar. *(a)* A plaque-induced periodontal lesionis seen as loss of distal crestal bone along with the first signs of apical radiolucency. *(b)* Both lesions have enlarged, one advancing apically (crown-down) and the other coronally (down-crown). The lesions remain separate. *(c)* The two periodontal lesions of differing etiology have merged into a single large lesion. At this point, it is clinically impossible to accurately establish the exact extension of and division between the two original individual pathologies. *(d and e)* Clinical and radiologic evidence confirm, simultaneous apicomarginal periodontal disease, defining the lesion as endo-perio:

* Patient history
* Pocket depth of 12 mm and a configuration that begins broadly but narrows distinctly to a point where the probe sinks into a tract leading to the apex
* Lack of pulp vitality ascertained by negative responses to the full range of thermal, EPT, and cavity tests

Diagnosis: Class 3 combined endo-perio lesion

Figs 5-14f to 5-14j Endodontic treatment followed by restoration with tapered posts (ParaPost, Coltène) and composite resin.

Figs 5-14k to 5-14n *(k)* Three months posttreatment, the pocket depth was reduced from 12 mm to 6 mm. *(l)* RCT had eliminated the endodontic pathology, but the distal and interradicular pockets, secondary to periodontal disease, persisted. *(m and n)* Hemisection was performed[72] with particular emphasis on removing residual enamel spurs of the pulpal floor.

Figs 5-14a to 5-14e

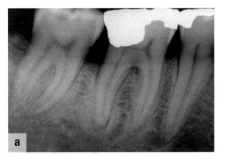

a

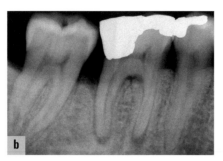

b

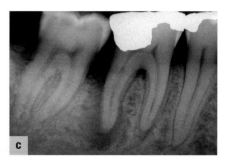

c

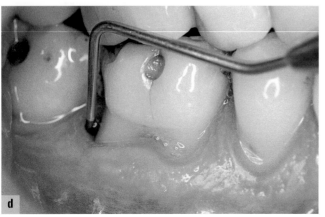

d

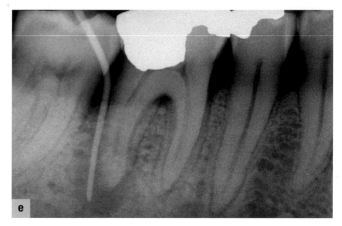

e

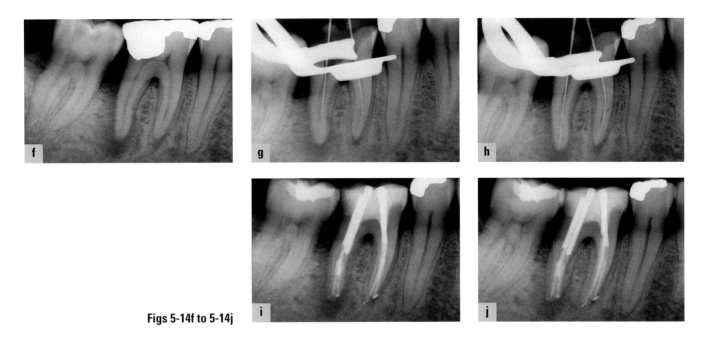

Figs 5-14f to 5-14j

Figs 5-14k to 5-14n

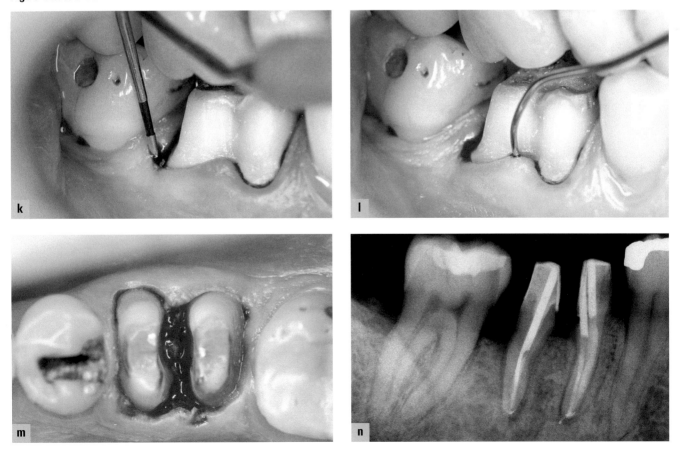

Figs 5-14o and 5-14p Hemisection eliminated the pocket at the furcation. The 5-mm distal pocket[43] and correction of the negative architecture[74,75] were then addressed.

Figs 5-14q to 5-14u Periodontal surgery included ostectomy along the coronal 3 mm of the intrabony defect[46] and guided bone regeneration with resorbable membrane[73] of the remaining 2 mm of the defect. (Courtesy of Dr Gianfranco Carnevale.)

Figs 5-14v to 5-14y *(v and w)* Four months after the periodontal treatment, the tissues are free of inflammation, probing depths are within 3 mm, and the negative architecture has been corrected. *(x and y)* Restoration with a metal-ceramic FPD to avoid sacrificing further dentin.

Figs 5-14z and 5-14aa Definitive posttreatment results.

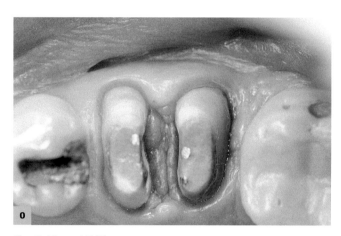
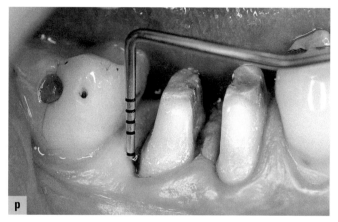

Figs 5-14o and 5-14p

Figs 5-14q to 5-14u

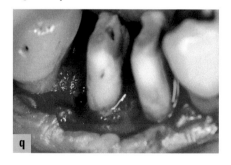
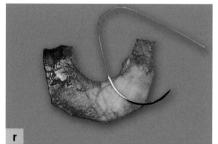
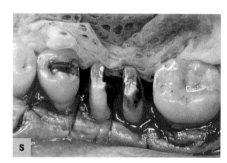

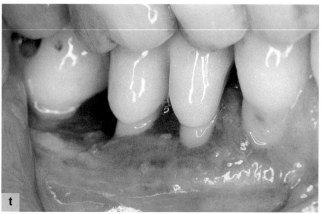
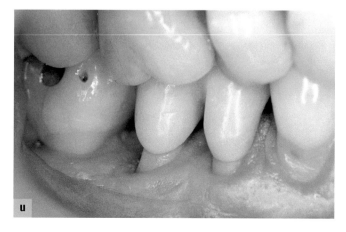

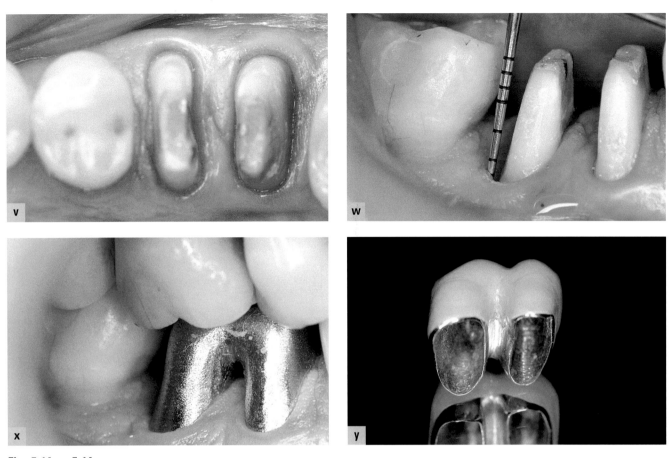

Figs 5-14v to 5-14y

Figs 5-14z and 5-14aa

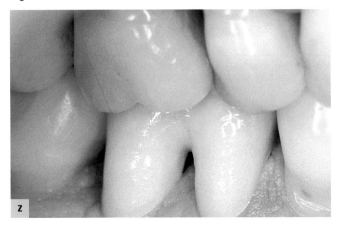

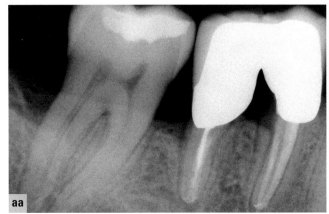

Sinus tract versus vertical root fracture: Clinical case studies 15 and 16

Probing into an isolated fissure does not necessarily indicate a draining sinus tract produced by endodontic pathology; it may also be secondary to vertical fracture or various anomalies of root anatomy. When first examined clinically these phenomena may be indistinguishable as their signs and symptoms can be identical. In many cases, a definitive diagnosis requires visual examination of the root by means of surgical exposure. When vertical root fracture is suspected the clinician must proceed with treatment cautiously until the diagnosis has been confirmed. Clinical case studies 15 and 16 illustrate this topic.

Clinical case study 15

Figs 5-15a to 5-15e A 50-year-old female patient presented with extensive previous endodontic therapy and restorations. *(a)* A well-defined appeared radiolucency at the apex of the mandibular left first premolar. This tooth had had previous RCT and cast post and core buildup and was the mesial abutment for a metal-ceramic FPD extending to the second molar. *(b to d)* Marginal recession of 3 mm was found and probing depths were within 3 mm. *(e)* An isolated area had a probing depth of 10 mm. One of the risks of a potential endo-perio profile with overall apicomarginal involvement is that a periodontal lesion limited to the buccal or palatal surface may not be visible radiologically because the root may camouflage the lesion.

Figs 5-15f to 5-15k An access flap revealed a vertical root fracture resulting in the extraction of the first premolar.

Figs 5-15a to 5-15e

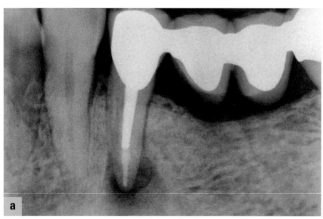

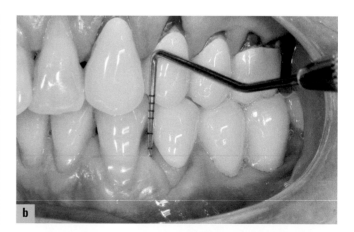

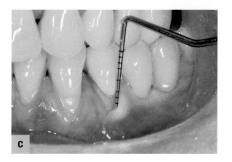

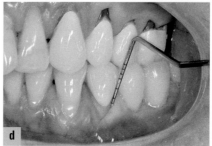

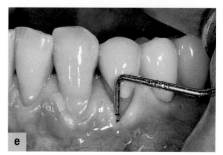

Figs 5-15f to 5-15k

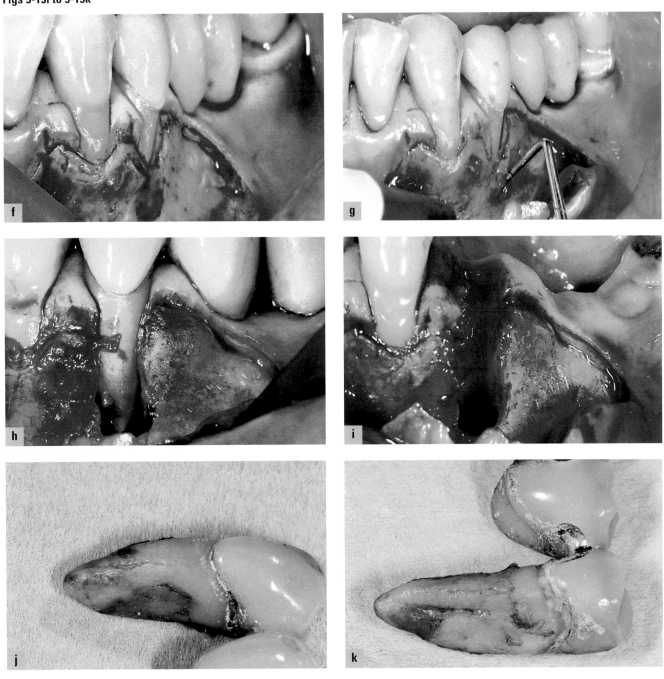

Clinical case study 16

Figs 5-16a to 5-16e A 40-year-old male patient presented with an endodontically treated mandibular left second premolar. *(a)* Extensive apical radiolucency surrounded the tooth. *(b to e)* As in case study 15, the probe located a single narrow defect. The patient's overall periodontal condition was fair. The patient's history of RCT and reasonably good periodontal health pointed to a diagnosis of Class 2 periodontal lesion of endodontic origin. A treatment plan of apicoectomy and step-back obturation was selected.

Figs 5-16f to 5-16k Stages of surgical endodontic treatment. Initial partial thickness marginal incision followed by full-thickness flap scalloping.

Figs 5-16a to 5-16e

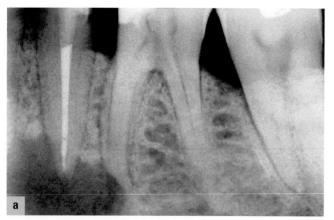
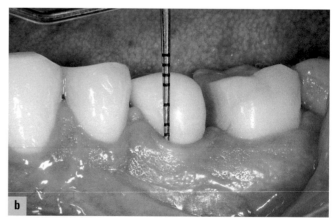

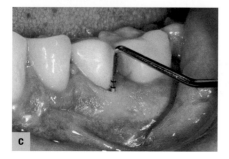
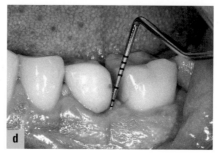
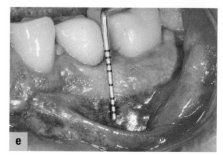

Figs 5-16f to 5-16k

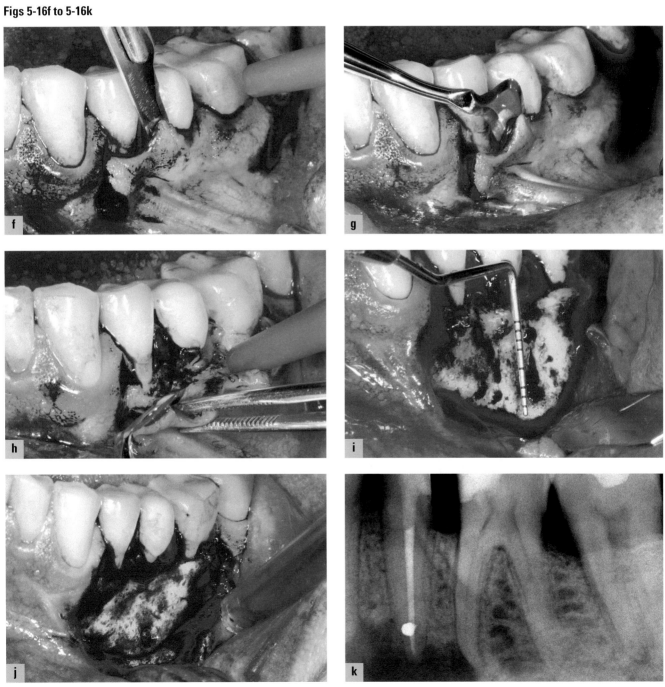

Figs 5-16l to 5-16r Further stages of surgical endodontic treatment. Ultrasonic surgical instruments (Easy Surgery [BioSaf]) were used because of the proximity of the inferior alveolar nerve.

Figs 5-16s to 5-16x *(s to u)* The retrograde cavity was prepared by step-back use of ultrasonic tips (Pro Ultra [Maillefer]) and sealed with MTA. *(v and w)* Observe the apical fragment removed and radiograph of the remaining root as evidence of the extent of the surgery. *(x)* The flap was closed with 4-0 silk sutures (Ethicon).

Figs 5-16y to 5-16bb *(y and z)* Follow-up at 6 months showing signs of satisfactory healing. Choice of incision and surgical technique reduced the risk of marginal gingival recession in the treatment area. *(aa and bb)* During the 13-month follow-up, rapidly progressing caries were detected at the distal margin of the second premolar *(white arrow)*. The caries, combined with remaining periodontal osseous defects *(red arrows)*, further complicated management of a challenging case.

Figs 5-16l to 5-16r

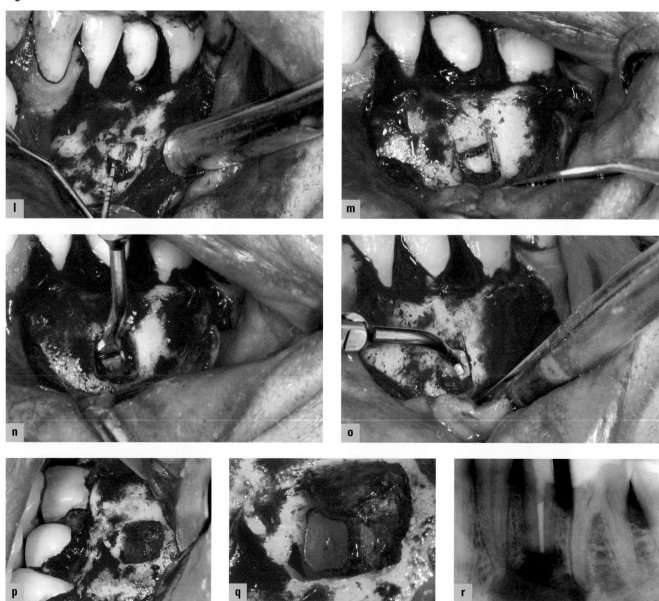

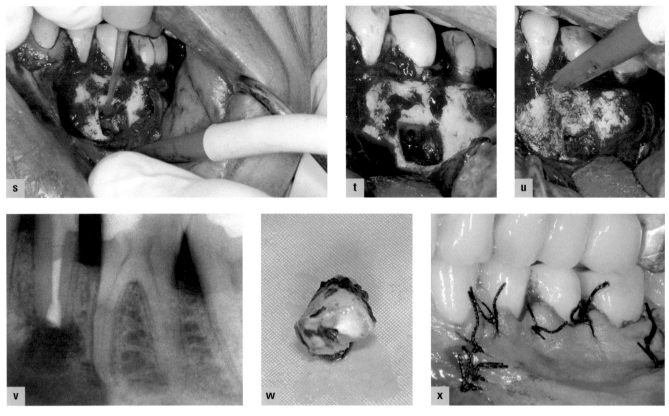

Figs 5-16s to 5-16x

Figs 5-16y to 5-16bb

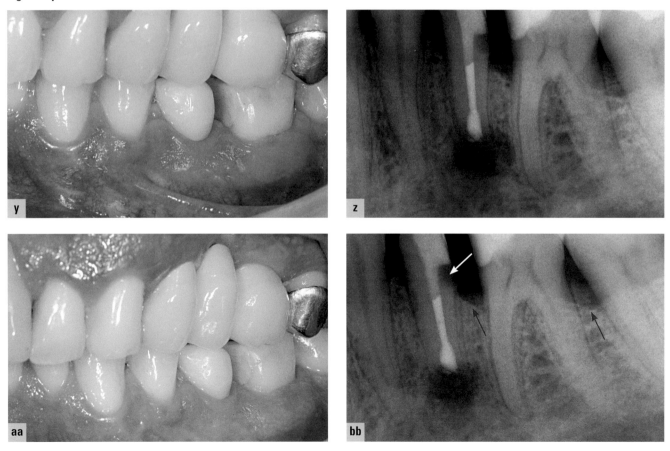

Figs 5-16cc to 5-16ee Periodontal assessment at the 13-month follow-up. The apicoectomy had eliminated the deep buccal defect associated with endodontic pathology but not the interproximal pockets associated with generalized chronic periodontitis. A new treatment plan included surgery to correct the persisting periodontal defects while allowing access to treat the caries that had spread along the distal margin of the second premolar.

Figs 5-16ff to 5-16kk *(ff to ii)* Incision and reflection of partial thickness flap on the buccal side. Osseous resective surgery followed by removal of carious dentin and placement of a composite restoration. Careful isolation of the area with rubber dam was vital to success. *(jj and kk)* Thinned buccal flap closed with sutures anchored to periosteum apical to the osseous crest. Observe the new relationship between gingival margin and provisional restoration.

Fig 5-16ll Three-week follow-up.

Figs 5-16cc to 5-16ee

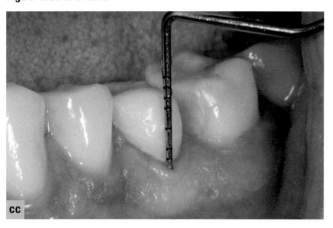

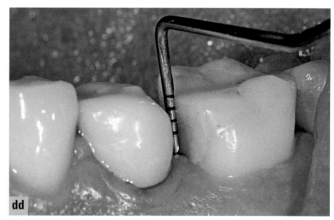

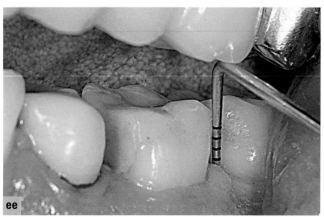

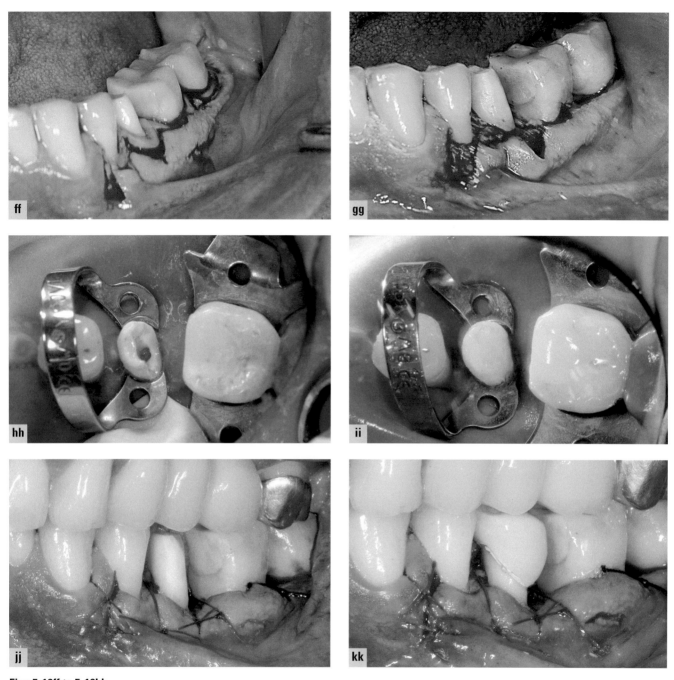

Figs 5-16ff to 5-16kk

Fig 5-16ll

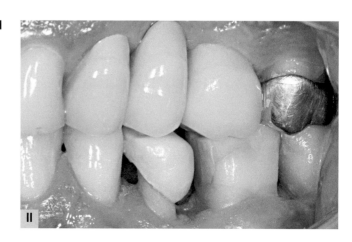

Clinical Case Study 17

Figs 5-17a to 5-17f Radiographs showed extensive loss of periodontal support surrounding the mandibular left first molar and the mesial aspect of the second molar. The overall picture was of very poor generalized periodontal health.

Preliminary differential diagnosis: Endo-perio profile

Periodontal assessment

Pocket width and depth was confirmed through radiographs showing evident bone loss and subgingival calculus.

Initial diagnostic hypothesis

In light of the intact crown on the first molar and the small restoration on the second molar, evidence of pulp vitality would suffice to exclude any consideration of Class 2 lesions, therefore establishing a pseudo endo-perio profile.

Conversely, any doubt as to pulp vitality would lead to assumption of an endo-perio profile, dictating the next dia-

Figs 5-17a to 5-17f

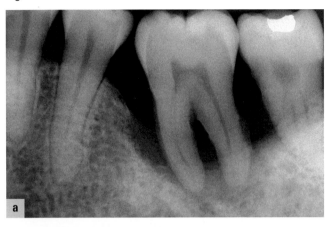

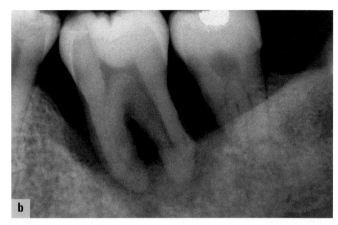

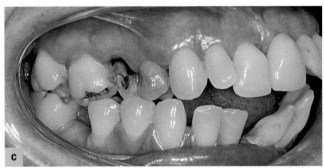

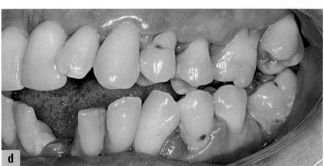

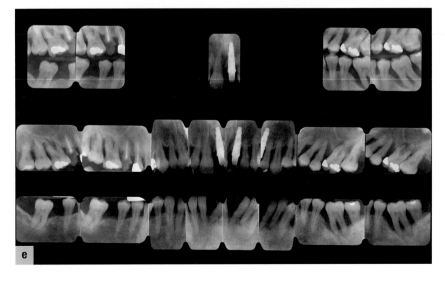

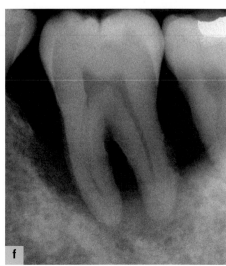

gnostic step: invasive cavity testing. If also negative, and confirmed by pulp nonresponse during root canal instrumentation, the pulp necrosis would signify that at least a portion of the apical lesion is of endodontic origin. If there is a vital reaction during instrumentation, as frequently occurs, it is possible that pulp necrosis has been caused by plaque pathogens entering the apex and damaging the pulp. It is plausible that this necrosis has in turn caused a further superimposed periodontal lesion. In this case, the diagnosis would be established as a Class 3 combined endo-perio lesion.

From a practical point of view, these ideas are of purely theoretical interest, not clinical relevance; they do not influence treatment decisions.

Figs 5-17g to 5-17k Cavity testing of the first and second molars was performed. *(g)* The first molar was nonresponsive to all vitality tests. *(h)* The second molar had a positive response when the bur entered the pulp chamber. The lack of pulp vitality in the first molar points to an endodontic factor contributing to the lesion in question. At a point in the future, this might be of clinical relevance if advances in regenerative surgery continue.[74] In the meantime, establishing the exact degree of pulp vitality in such cases does not affect the decision to proceed with extraction. *(i to k)* The extracted first molar had extensive deposits of plaque and calculus from crown to apex.

Figs 5-17g to 5-17k

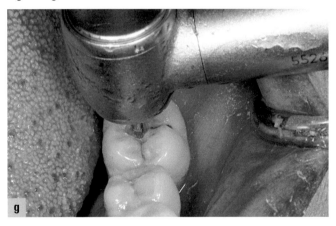

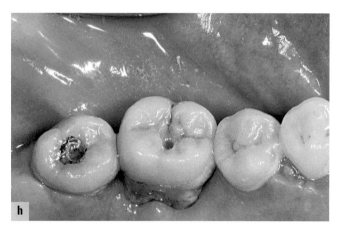

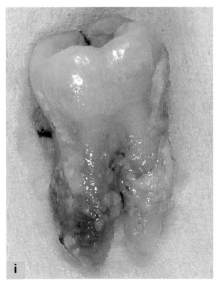

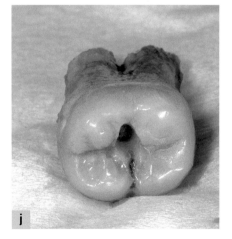

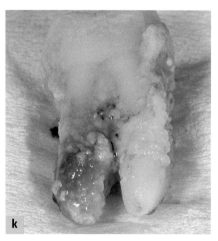

Clinical case study 18

Figs 5-18a and 5-18b A 57-year-old male patient presented with a sinus tract draining on the buccal side of his mandibular left second molar. Clinical and radiologic examinations indicate overall apicomarginal periodontal involvement. There was no response to vitality tests including cavity testing.

Figs 5-18c to 5-18f Logic associates this lesion with pulp necrosis. *(c)* The crown has a crack extending from the base of the pulp cavity along its distal wall *(black arrow). (d)* The periodontal situation elsewhere is fair, but probing depth at the mesial of this second molar was 9 mm. In addition, the sinus tract at first observation appeared to be intrasulcular but is in fact is paramarginal *(white arrows)*.

Figs 5-18a and 5-18b

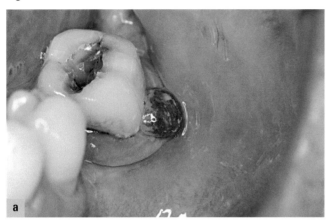 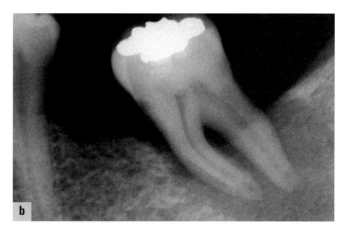

Figs 5-18c to 5-18f

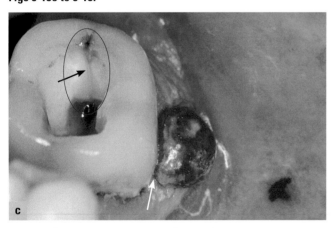 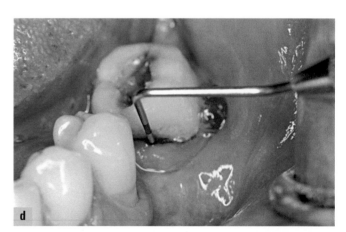

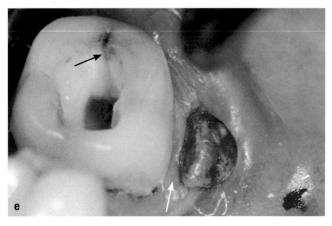 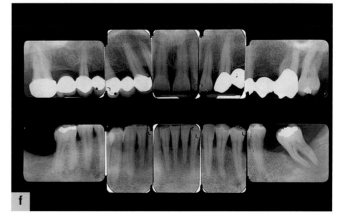

Diagnosis: Class 2 periodontal lesion of endodontic origin

Conjecturally, the same lesion minus the 9-mm pocket (implying an intact attachment apparatus) would be categorized as a pseudo Class 2 endo-perio lesion.

Figs 5-18g to 5-18k Stages of endodontic treatment are shown below. Apical resorption had occurred at the distal root, preventing an ideal apical seal, as confirmed by sealant leakage visible radiologically. Following RCT, symptoms improved immediately and the sinus tract disappeared.

Figs 5-18g to 5-18k

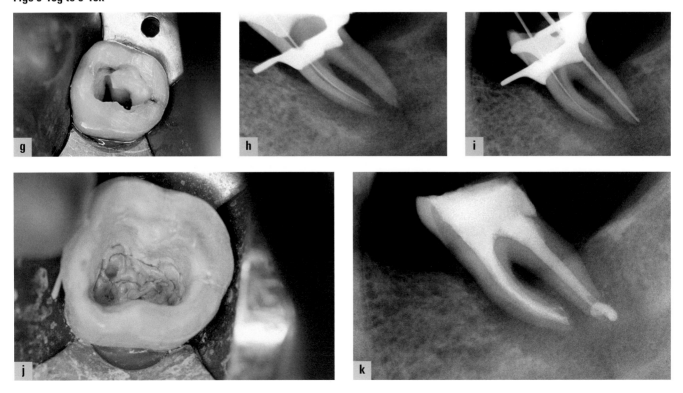

Figs 5-18l to 5-18p *(l to p)* Three months after completion of the endodontic treatment another sinus tract erupted distal to the same second molar *(arrows)*. The sinus tract was traced to a point near the distal root apex. Despite overall bone loss, probing depths were not excessive. The periodontal component could be excluded from the diagnosis.

Diagnosis: Class 2 pseudo endo-perio profile

Figs 5-18q to 5-18t Despite the extensive osseous defect, the tooth had good marginal support, and the patient opted for endodontic surgery.

Figs 5-18u to 5-18y At 6-month *(u to w)* and 12-month *(x and y)* follow-ups, there is radiologic evidence of periradicular healing and an absence of excessive probing depths.

Figs 5-18l to 5-18p

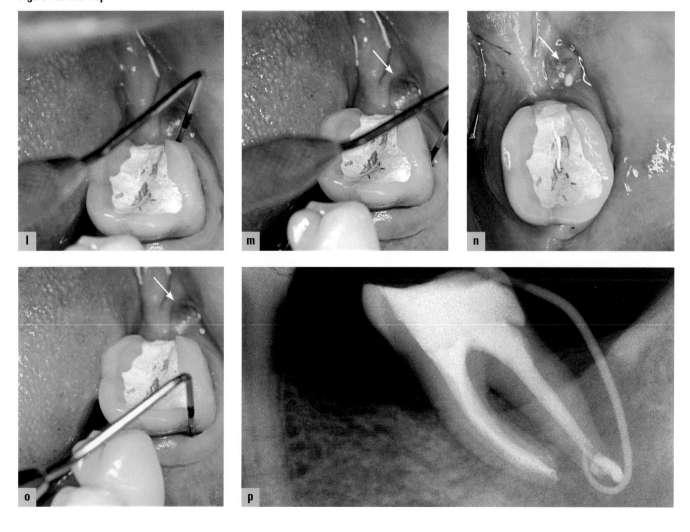

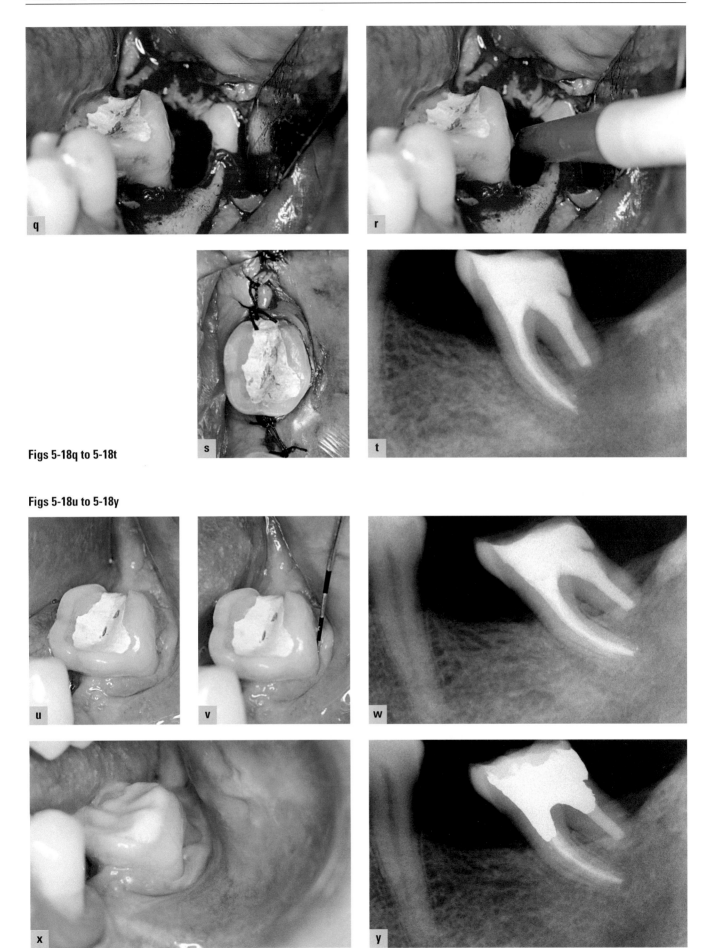

Figs 5-18q to 5-18t

Figs 5-18u to 5-18y

Figs 5-18z to 5-18cc Pre- and posttreatment records. Diagnoses were a Class 2 endo-perio lesion affecting the mesial root, followed by a Class 2 pseudo endo-perio lesion at the distal root.

Figs 5-18z to 5-18cc

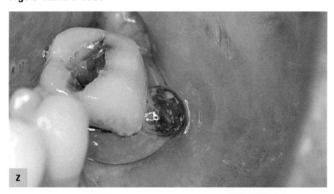

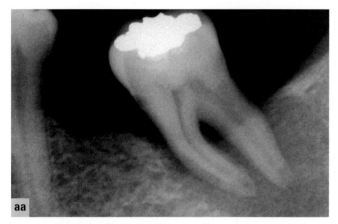

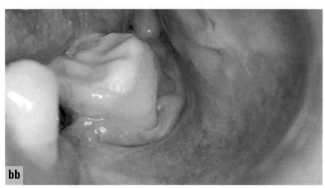

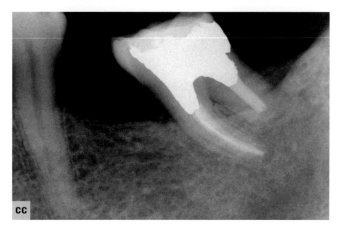

Clinical case study 19

Preliminary diagnosis: Endo-perio profile

Figs 5-19a and 5-19b *(a)* A 55-year-old female, previously treated for a malignant tumor but currently cancer-free, presents with swelling buccal to the mandibular right first molar. Although treated endodontically, the mesial root canal was lacking an adequate seal against influx of pathogens. *(b)* Radiographs showed a radiolucency extending from the mesial root towards the furcation, indicating a Class II furcation invasion. Probing depth was 12 mm with copious bleeding on probing.

Figs 5-19c and 5-19d A gutta-percha point inserted into the sulcus indicated the mesial root apex as the origin of a sinus tract. Combined with findings upon probing and general good periodontal health, the furcation involvement suggested an endodontic source for the defect. However, further investigation was required to eliminate fracture, perforation, and periodontal factors as contributors to this lesion. Direct visualization by means of exploratory flap surgery was needed to complete the diagnosis.

Figs 5-19a and 5-19b

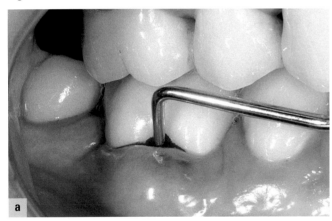
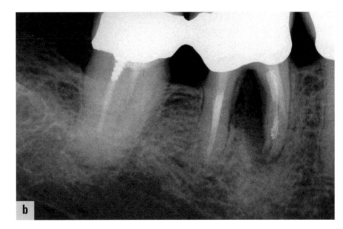

Figs 5-19c and 5-19d

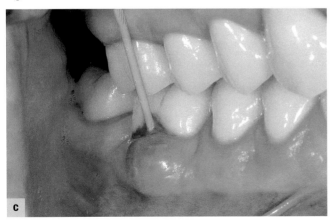
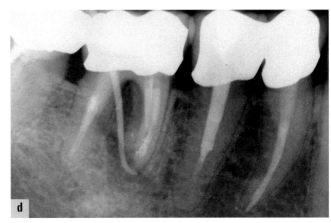

Figs 5-19e to 5-19h Access flap reflected and granulation tissue removed so as to appreciate the extent of the lesion.

Figs 5-19i to 5-19l The mesial root was uncovered and its apex accessed with surgical ultrasonic tips (Easy Surgery [BioSaf]). In the absence of signs of fracture, perforation, or stripping damage, the mesial root was prepared for apicoectomy. The apex was resected, instrumented, and stepback sealed with MTA.

Figs 5-19e to 5-19h

Figs 5-19i to 5-19l

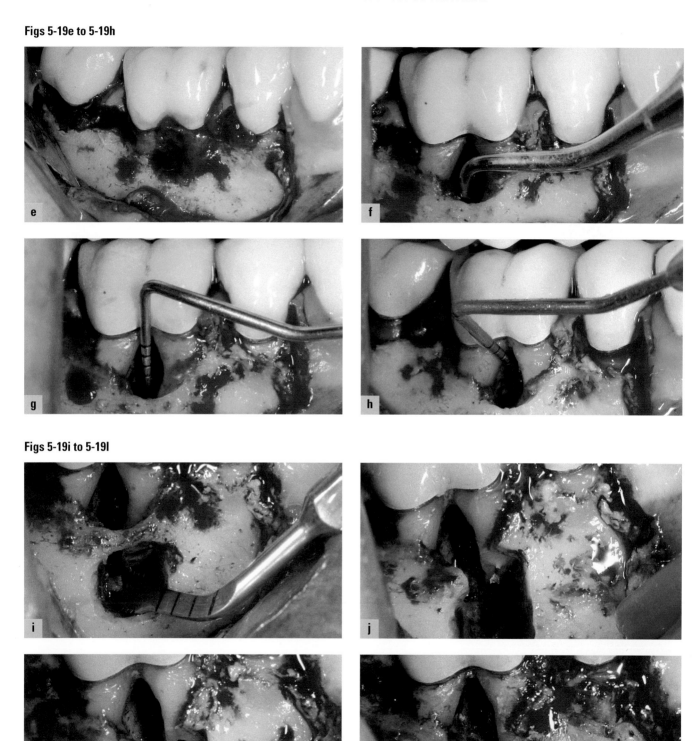

Figs 5-19m to 5-19o Close-up images of the apex. *(m)* Inadequate obturation, allowing bacterial infiltration *(white arrow)*. *(n)* Cavity preparation with ultrasonic tips. *(o)* Step-back cavity sealing with MTA.[75,76]

Figs 5-19p to 5-19s *(p)* The bony defect and surgical site filled with osteoconductive grafting material and covered with a resorbable collagen membrane. *(q and r)* The gingiva were closed with 5-0 Vicryl sutures (Ethicon). *(s)* Postoperative control radiograph.

Figs 5-19m to 5-19o

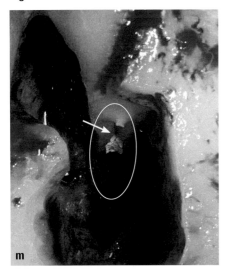
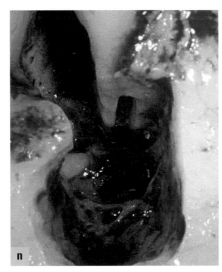
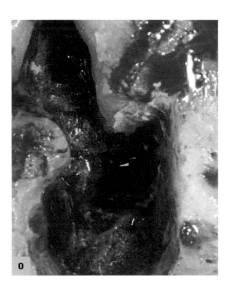

Figs 5-19p to 5-19s

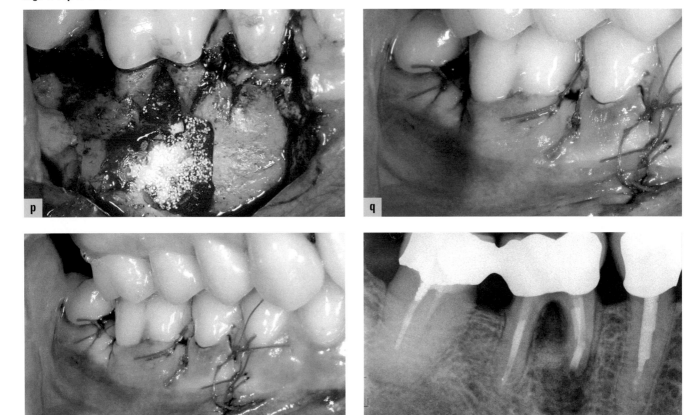

Figs 5-19t to 5-19aa Posttreatment records at 3 months *(t and u)*, 6 months *(v and w)*, 8 months *(x and y)*, and 14 months *(z and aa)* showing visible evidence of progressive healing. A pronounced furcation defect persists although its probing depth is acceptable. Maintaining good hygiene in this area is challenging for the patient, but clinical signs of inflammation are not apparent.

Figs 5-19t to 5-19aa

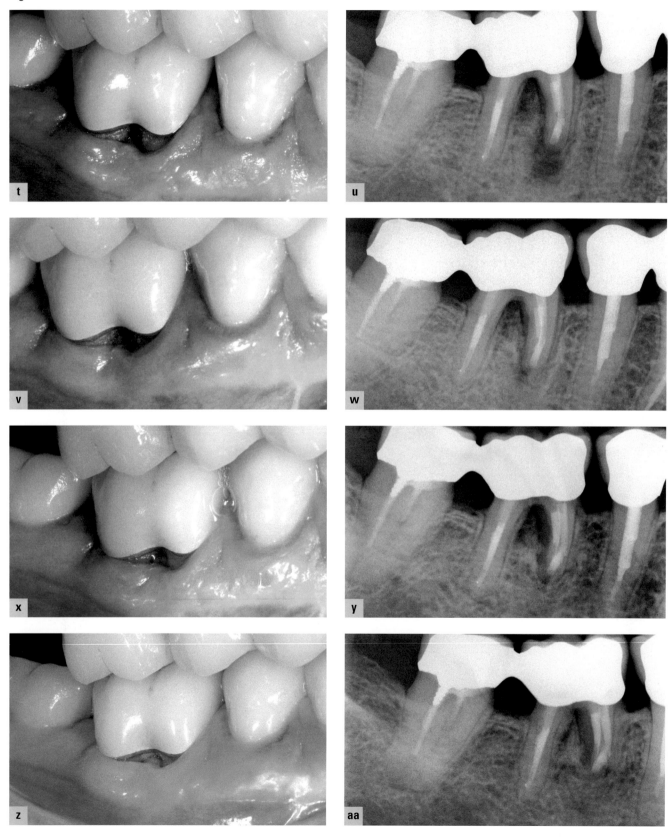

Clinical case study 20

Figs 5-20a to 5-20d *(a and b)* The patient presented with a sinus tract draining mesiolingual *(white arrow)* to the mandibular right second premolar. This tooth is the mesial abutment for a metal-ceramic FPD with the right second molar as the distal abutment and mesial cantilevers to replace the right first premolar. *(c)* The second premolar has been treated endodontically and restored with a cast post and core. The mesial end of the FPD is mobile. *(d)* There is a radiolucent area extending along the length of the mesial aspect of the root *(red arrows)* but no appreciable apical radiolucency.

Figs 5-20a to 5-20d

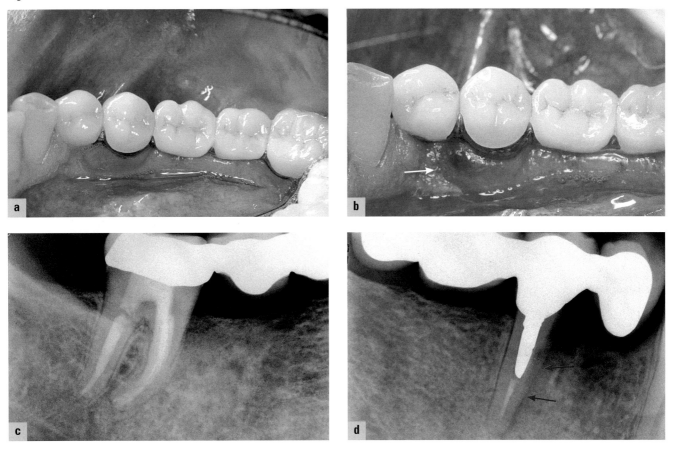

Figs 5-20e to 5-20h The FPD was dislodged from its distal abutment, allowing its removal. The cast post and core was no longer cemented to the second premolar and was removed as one piece with the FPD.

Figs 5-20i to 5-20m *(i to m)* Circumferential probing of the sulcus was within normal limits (3 mm) until probing the mesiolingual line angle, where the probe located a 10-mm pocket. The apical aspect of this pocket was narrow.

Figs 5-20e to 5-20h

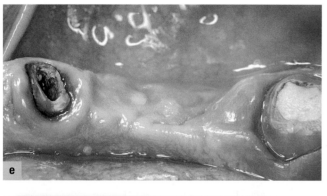

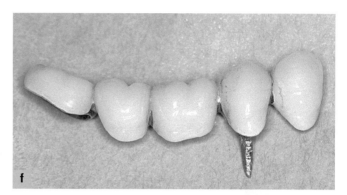

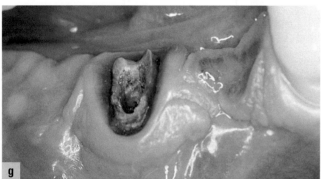

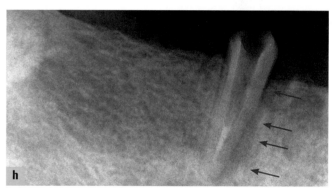

Figs 5-20i to 5-20m

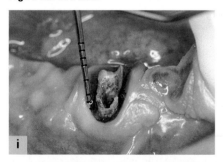

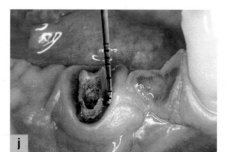

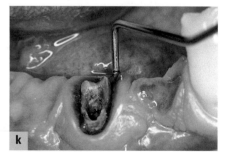

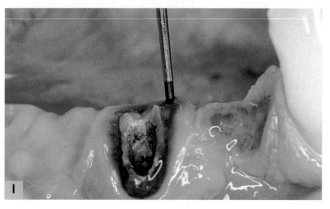

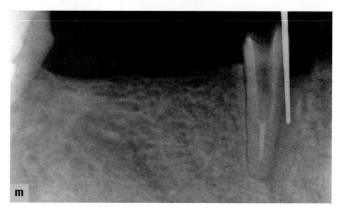

Figs 5-20n to 5-20p A radiograph taken with a gutta-percha point inserted into the pocket confirmed the presence of a defect extending just short of the apex. Vertical root fracture of the second premolar was suspected based on a number of factors: *(1)* previous RCT and post and core preparation had removed substantial tooth structure; *(2)* the cantilever end of the FPD is adjacent to the premolar; *(3)* probing depths are shallow with the exception of one distinct intra-

bony defect; and *(4)* patient history reveals earlier root fracture of the right first premolar. Because the treatment for root fracture is extraction, such a diagnosis must be confirmed beyond reasonable doubt, preferably by means of direct visual inspection. Prior to resorting to an access flap, a nonsurgical approach to diagnosis continued.

Figs 5-20q to 5-20s The tooth is isolated, original gutta-percha filling removed, and the canal disinfected.

Figs 5-20n to 5-20p

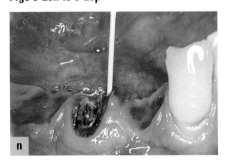
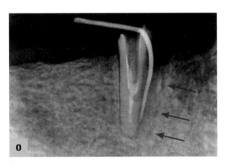
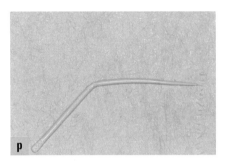

Figs 5-20q to 5-20s

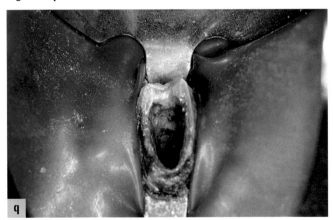
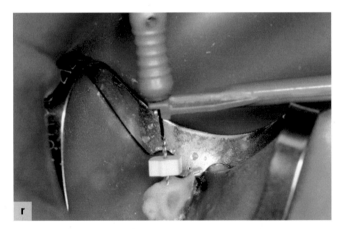

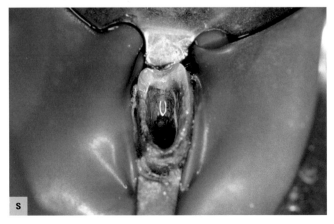

Figs 5-20t to 5-20w *(t to u)* A 0.6-caliber curved instrument was inserted into a lateral canal *(arrow)* which had not been located or treated previously. Previous radiologic evidence aided in locating this canal. *(v and w)* Radiopaque sealer and gutta-percha filling highlighted the path of the lateral canal *(arrow)*.

Preliminary diagnosis: Class 2 down-crown lesion secondary to lateral canal vs Class 3 combined endo-perio lesion

Fig 5-20x After completion of endodontic retreatment, the cast post and core and FPD are recemented.

Figs 5-20t to 5-20w

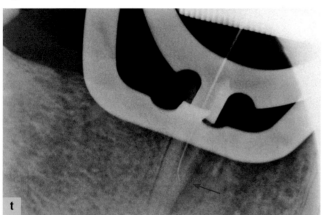
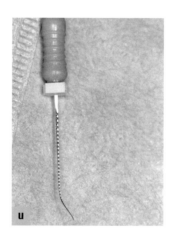
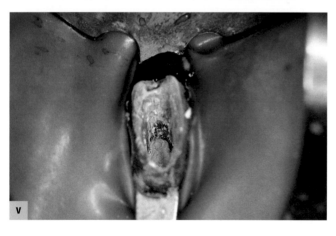
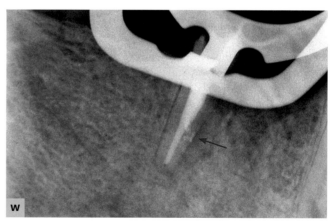

Fig 5-20x

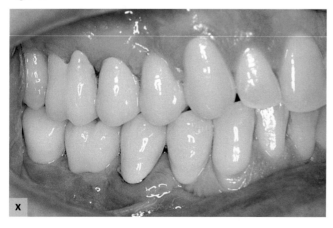

Figs 5-20y to 5-20bb After 1 week, the sinus tract closed and had not reappeared when the patient presented for the 3-month follow-up appointment.

Figs 5-20cc to 5-20gg *(cc)* After six months posttreatment the second premolar has clearly improved. *(dd and ee)* A remaining 5-mm pocket was assumed to be a consequence of a secondary periodontitis. This defect was addressed with localized periodontal scaling and root planing. *(ff and gg)* One- and two-year posttreatment records confirm further improvement.

Final diagnosis: Class 3 combined endo-perio lesion

Figs 5-20y to 5-20bb

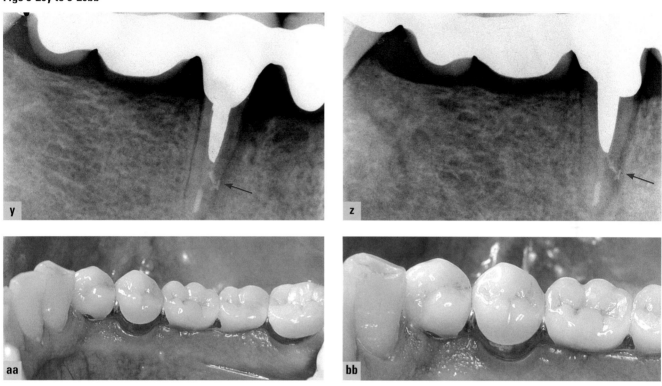

Figs 5-20cc to 5-20gg

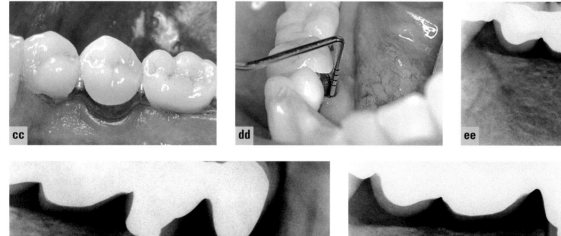

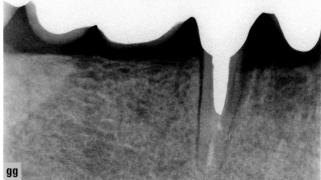

Figs 5-20hh to 5-20ll Four-year posttreatment records attested to a stable condition: minimal periodontal inflammation, good tissue adaptation to root surfaces, and a pocket depth of 3 mm at the site of the old lesion.

Considerations

A temporary return to the five-part endo-perio classification system of Simon, Glick, and Frank[2] will provide an interesting context for analysis of this case. Three of their proposed categories can be applied:

Primary endodontic lesion

A primary endodontic lesion became a viable option when the lateral canal was discovered because it indicated a potential sinus tract emerging in the sulcus. However, the residual 5-mm probing depth after endodontic treatment forced consideration of further alternative diagnostic hypotheses.

Primary endodontic lesion with secondary periodontal involvement

A primary endodontic lesion with secondary periodontal involvement is plausible because the sinus tract orifice in the sulcus permits the entrance of bacteria and colonization of the root surface, leading to a plaque-induced periodontal lesion. Once RCT has resolved the endodontic component, the plaque-induced periodontal condition remains, as confirmed by residual marginal pocket depths.

Combined endo-perio lesion

A combined endo-perio lesion is possible if a genuine periodontal pocket began marginally concurrent to apical sinus tract formation.

In any case, it is impossible to ascertain if the source of the residual pocket was a periodontal infection secondary to a sinus tract or was a preexisting condition that itself contributed to the emergence of the sinus tract. The clinical approach would not vary: endodontic treatment, a period of healing, periodontal reassessment, and periodontal treatment as necessary.

Figs 5-20hh to 5-20ll

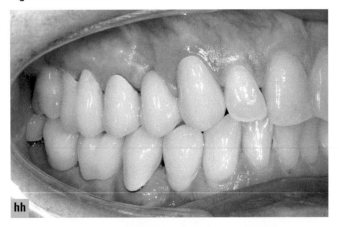

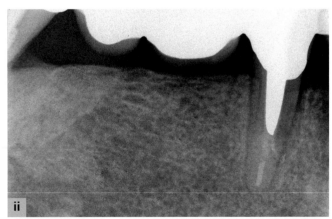

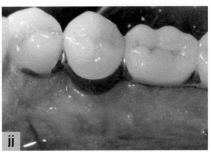

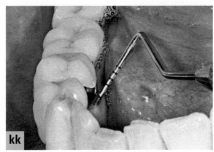

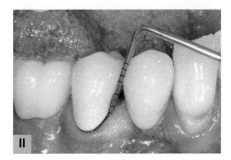

Clinical case study 21

Figs 5-21a and 5-21b A 64-year old male patient presented with a complaint of localized "tightness," swelling, and inflammation in the area of a 3-unit FPD that connects the maxillary right canine to the second premolar. The premolar distal abutment was mobile. The canine was stable, but its unit of the FPD had debonded. *(a)* Direct examination revealed a fracture in the exposed dentin at the cervical margin of the FPD *(green circle)*. *(b)* Radiologic examination showed considerable bone loss, especially towards the mesial side of the second premolar *(left arrows)*. There was also a modest area of radiolucency around the root of the canine *(right arrow)*. Poor marginal fit of the FPD was also noted *(circle)*.

Figs 5-21c to 5-21g *(c to e)* In spite of lack of mobility, the canine did have an isolated pocket depth of 8 mm adjacent to the observed midbuccal fracture line. *(f)* The second premolar was very mobile with generalized loss of attachment culminating in a deep pocket towards the mesial. *(g)* Probing chart for this quadrant. Despite inadequate hygiene, no other probing depths exceeded 3 mm. The premolar was responsive to pulp vitality tests but the canine was not.

Figs 5-21a and 5-21b

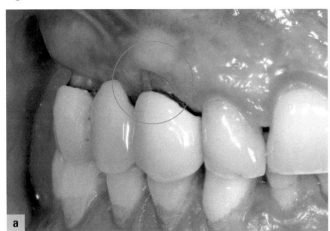 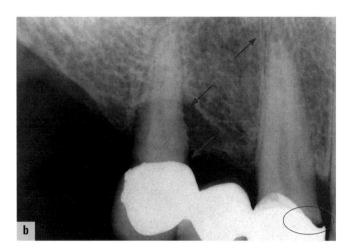

Figs 5-21c to 5-21g

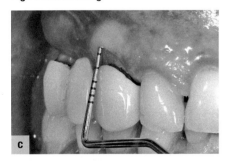 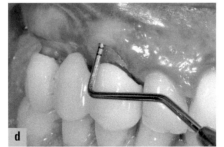 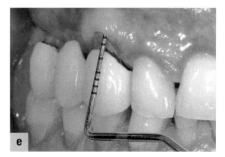

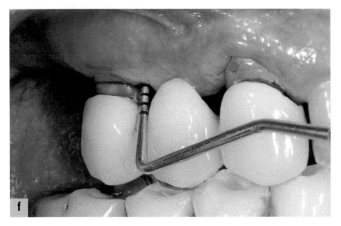

16	15	14	13	12	11
	658		282	222	323
	6710		222	222	323
	3		3?		
	3		3		

Figs 5-21h to 5-21k The FPD was sectioned and removed from the canine abutment, revealing an oblique tooth fracture at the distobuccal line angle that extended 1 mm apical to the gingival margin *(arrows)*.

Figs 5-21l to 5-21o The fractured segment did not affect the tooth's attachment apparatus, as evidenced by probing depths within normal limits in the adjacent sulcus. The isolated midbuccal pocket was remeasured at 9 mm in the absence of the FPD.

Figs 5-21h to 5-21k

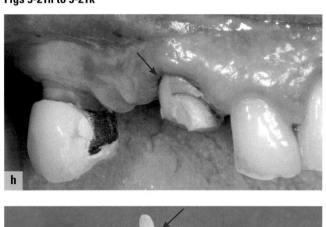

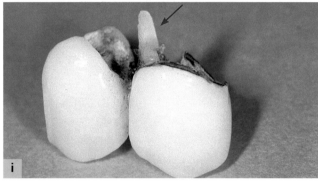

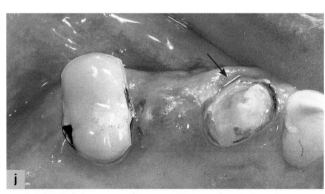

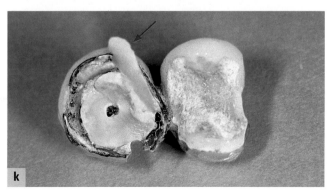

Figs 5-21l to 5-21o

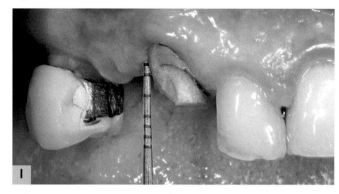

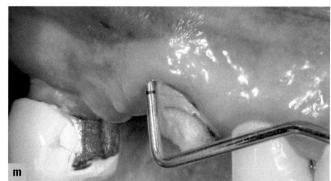

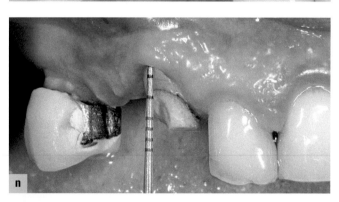

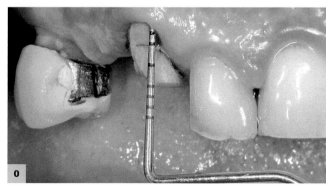

Figs 5-21p to 5-21s Probing depths around the second premolar were consistent with the broad pocket configuration of a Class 1 lesion. Despite the presence of pockets and mobility, the gingival appearance and modest bleeding on repeated probing did not indicate acute inflammation of this area.

Figs 5-21t to 5-21w The stages of RCT and provisional restoration are shown. Opening the pulp cavity of the canine revealed necrotic pulp.

Figs 5-21p to 5-21s

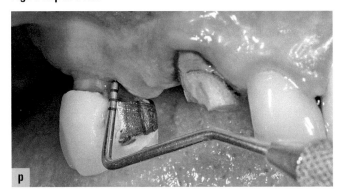

Figs 5-21t to 5-21w

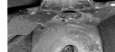

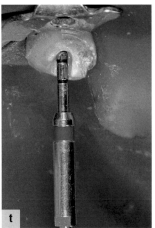

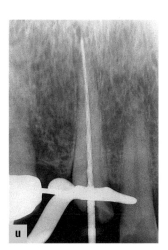

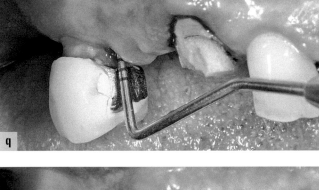

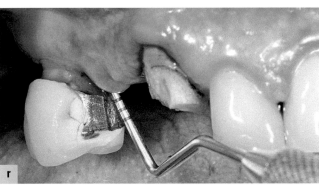

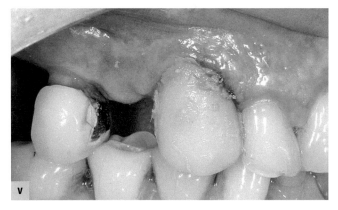

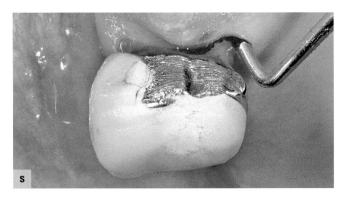

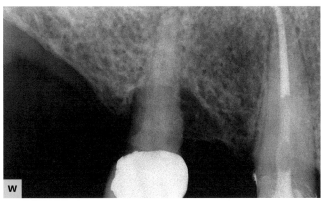

Figs 5-21x and 5-21y After 1 week, the canine exhibited reduced gingival inflammation and improved probing depths. The second premolar remained problematic despite scaling and root planing during the endodontic treatment. At the next follow-up, a decision was made to extract this tooth in light of its poor prognosis and to proceed with implant-supported restorations.

Figs 5-21z to 5-21ff *(z and aa)* Extraction of the second premolar and postextraction surgical decontamination of the alveolar site.[77] *(bb to ff)* widening of the alveolar crest with a ridge-splitting technique and simultaneous insertion of implants[18,78–80] (Exacta, Biaggini). *(cc)* Flap reflection allows direct visualization of the canine alveolus with no signs of vertical root fracture.

Figs 5-21x and 5-21y

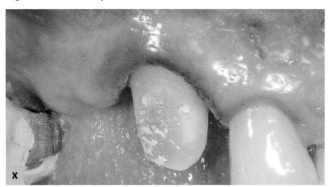

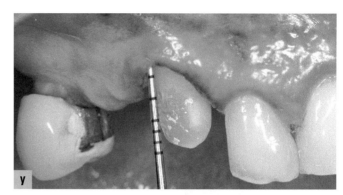

Figs 5-21z to 5-21ff

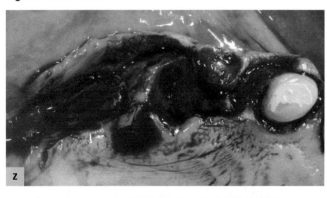

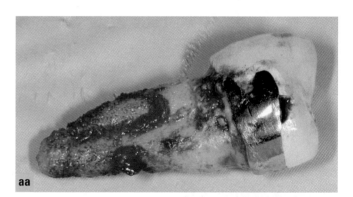

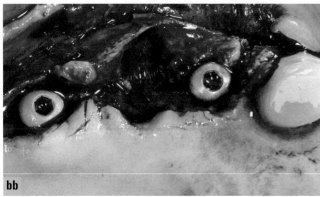

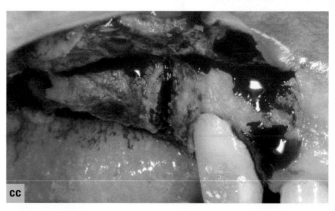

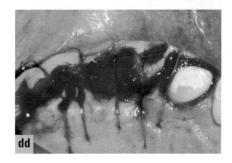

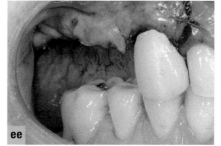

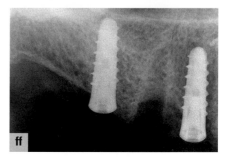

Figs 5-21gg to 5-21kk The final stages of multidisciplinary endodontic-surgical-implant rehabilitation are shown below. Observe the correct crest profile, positioning, and angle of implant abutments. Marginal tissues surrounding the canine are free of signs of inflammation and show good adaptation to the restoration.

This case is a prime example of the importance of careful, unhurried evaluation of all clinical evidence. A hasty, insufficiently confirmed diagnosis of canine root fracture would have radically altered the treatment plan. The complexity of endo-perio lesions is fraught with traps into which the clinician can sadly fall. A thorough investigation based on a competent, pragmatic approach is a duty to both patients and profession. ◾

Figs 5-21gg to 5-21kk

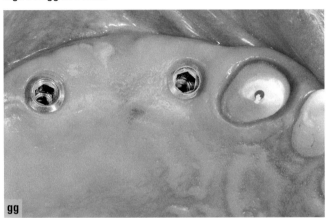

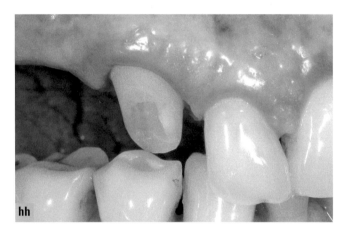

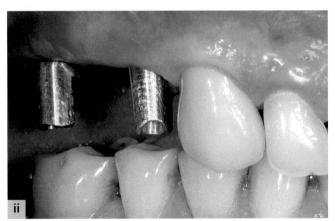

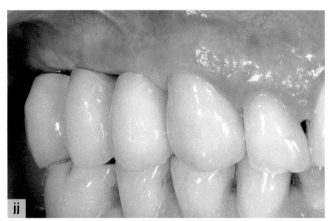

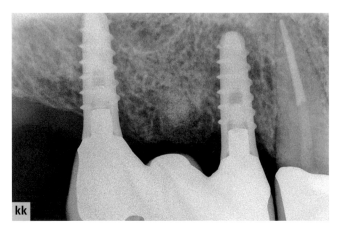

Bibliography

1. Barboni MG, Zucchelli G. Le relazioni endodontico-parodontali. Quaderni Clinici. Milan: Società Italiana di Endodonzia, 2006.

2. Simon JHS, Glick DH, Frank AL. The relationship of endodontic-periodontic lesions. J Periodontol 1972;43:202–208.

3. Torabinejad M. Endodontic-periodontic interrelationships. In: Walton RE, Torabinejad M (eds). Principles and Practice of Endodontics. Philadelphia: Saunders, 1989:433–446.

4. Vignoletti, G. Le relazioni endo-parodontali. G Ital Endod 1989;2(3):27.

5. Bergenholtz G, Hasselgren G. Endodonzia e parodontologia. In: Lindhe J (ed). Parodontologia e Implantologia Dentale, ed 3. Milan: Ermes, 1998:300–305.

6. Castellucci A. Endodonzia. Prato: Tridente, 1993.

7. Hiatt WH. Pulpal periodontal disease. J Periodontol 1977;48:598–609.

8. Pecora G, Kim S. Advanced endodontic microsurgery. Presented at the 54th Annual Session of the American Association of Endodontists, Seattle, 7–10 May 1998.

9. Bender IB, Seltzer S. The effect of periodontal disease on the pulp. Oral Surg Oral Med Oral Pathol 1972;33:458–474.

10. Eco U. Il nome della rosa. Milan: Bompiani, 1980.

11. Everet FG, Kramer GM. The distolingual groove in the maxillary lateral incisor: A periodontal hazard. J Periodontol 1972;43:352–361.

12. Withers JA, Brunsvold MA, Killoy WJ, Rahe AJ. The relationship of palato-gingival grooves to localized periodontal disease. J Periodontol 1981;52:41–44.

13. Frank AL. External-internal progressive resorption and its nonsurgical correction. J Endod 1981;7:473.

14. Heithersay GS. Invasive cervical resorption: an analysis of potential predisposing factors. Quintessence Int 1999;30:83–95.

15. Marcoli PA, Pizzi S, Righi D. I riassorbimenti invasivi cervicali, III: Trattamento e casi clinici. G Ital Endod 2001;3:108–114.

16. Marcoli PA, Pizzi S, Righi D. I riassorbimenti radicolari, I: Rassegna della letteratura. G Ital Endod 2001;1:8–14.

17. Lekovic V, Kenney EB, Weinlaender M, et al. A bone regenerative approach to alveolar ridge maintenance following tooth extraction. Report of 10 cases. J Periodontol 1997;68:563–570.

18. Scipioni A, Bruschi GB, Calesini G. The edentulous ridge expansion technique: A five-year study. Int J Periodontics Restorative Dent 1994;14:451–459.

19. Gargiulo AW, Wentz FFM, Orban B. Dimension of the dento-gingival junction in humans. J Periodontol 1961;32:261.

20. Maynard JG Jr, Wilson RD. Physiologic dimensions of the periodontium significant to the restorative dentist. J Periodontol 1979;50:170–174.

21. Parma-Benfenati S, Fugazzotto PA, Ruben MP. The effect of restorative margins on the postsurgical development and nature of the periodontium. Part 1. Int J Periodontics Restorative Dent 1985;5(6):30–51.

22. Vacek J, Gher M, Assad D, Richardson AC, Giambarresi L. The dimensions of the human dentogingival junction. Int J Periodontics Restorative Dent 1994;14:154–165.

23. Reeh ES, Messer HH, Douglas WH. Reduction in tooth stiffness as a result of endodontic and restorative procedures. J Endod 1989;15:512–516.

24. Renson CE. Elastic and mechanical properties of dentin [abstract]. J Dent Res 1968;47:992.

25. Testori T, Badino M, Castagnola M. Rassegna della letteratura internazionale sull'eziologia delle fratture verticali di radice. G Ital Endod 1990;4(3):44–47.

26. Trope M, Maltz DO, Tronstad L. Resistance to fracture of restored endodontically treated teeth. Endod Dent Traumatol 1985;1:108–111.

27. Seltzer S, Bender IB, Ziontz M. The interrelationship of pulp and periodontal disease. Oral Surg Oral Med Oral Pathol 1963;16:1474–1490.

28. Andreasen JO, Andreasen FM. Essentials of Traumatic Injuries to the Teeth. Copenhagen: Munksgaard, 1991.

29. Andersson L, Bodin I, Sorensen S. Progression of root resorption following replantation of human teeth after extended extraoral storage. Endod Dent Traumatol 1989;5:38–47.

30. Tronstad L, Andreasen JO, Hasselgren G, Kristerson L, Riis I. pH changes in dental tissues following root canal filling with calcium hydroxide. J Endod 1981;7:17–21.

31. Massarstrom LE, Blomlof LB, Feiglin B, Lindskog SF. Effect of calcium hydroxide treatment on periodontal repair and root resorption. Endod Dent Traumatol 1986;2:184–189.

32. Vertucci FJ, Williams RG. Furcation canals in the human mandibular first molar. J Oral Surg Oral Med Oral Pathol 1974;38:308–314.

33. Lowman JV, Burke RS, Pelleu GB. Patent accessory canals: Incidence in molar furcation region. Oral surg Oral Med Oral Pathol 1973;36:580–584.

34. Gutmann JL. Prevalence, location and patency of accessory canals in the furcation region of permanent molars. J Periodont 1978;49:21–26.

35. Burch JG, Hulen S. A study of the presence of accessory foramina and the topography of molar furcations. Oral Surg Oral Med Oral Pathol 1974;38:451–455.

36. Perlich MA, Reader A, Foreman DW. A scanning electron microscopic investigation of accessory foramens on the pulpal floor of human molars. J Endodon 1981;7:402–406.

37. De Deus QD. Frequency, location, and direction of the lateral, secondary, and accessory canals. J Endod 1975;1:361–366.

38. Grossman LI, Oliet S, Del Rio CE. Endodontic Practice, ed 11. Philadelphia: Lea & Febiger, 1988.

39. Torabinejad M, Walton RE, Ogilvie AL. Periapical pathosis. In: Ingle JI (ed). Endodontics, ed 3. Philadelphia: Lea & Febiger, 1985.

40. Schilder H. Nonsurgical endodontics. Presented at Goldman School of Dental Medicine, Boston University, Boston, 1978.

41. Jansson L, Ehnevid H, Lindskog S, Blomlöf L. Relationship between periapical and periodontal status. A clinical retrospective study. J Clin Periodontol 1993;20:117–123.

42. Corbet EF. Diagnosis of acute periodontal lesions. Periodontol 2000 2004;34:204–216.

43. Armitage GC. Periodontal diseases: diagnosis. Ann Periodontol 1996;1:37–215.

44. Kaldhal W, Kalkwarf KL, Patil KD, Molvar MP, Dyer JK. Long-term evaluation of periodontal therapy, I: Response to 4 therapeutic modalities. J Periodontol 1996;67:93–108.

45. Olsen C, Ammons W, van Belle G. A longitudinal study comparing apically repositioned flaps, with and without osseous surgery. Int J Periodontics Restorative Dent 1985;5(4):10–33.

46. Carnevale GF, Kaldahl W. Osseous resective surgery. Periodontol 2000 2000;22:59–87.

47. Carnevale G, Cordioli G, Mazzocco C, Brugnolo C. La tecnica della conservazione delle fibre gengivali. Dent Cadmos 1985;53(19):15–40.

48. Carnevale G. Fibre retention osseous resective surgery: A novel conservative approach for pocket elimination. J Clin Periodontol 2007;34:182–187.

49. Carnevale G, Sterrantino S, Di Febo G. Soft and hard tissue wound healing following tooth preparation to the alveolar crest. Int J Periodontics Restorative Dent 1983;3(6):36–53.

50. Carnevale GF, Di Febo GF, Biscaro L, Sterrantino SF, Fuzzi M. An in vivo study of teeth reprepared during periodontal surgery. Int J Periodontics Restorative Dent 1990;10:40–55.

51. Mazur B, Massler M. Influence of periodontal disease on the dental pulp. Oral Surg Oral Med Oral Pathol 1964;17:592–603.

52. Czarnecki RT, Schilder H. A histological evaluation of the human pulp in teeth with varying degrees of periodontal disease. J Endod 1979;5:242–253.

53. Torabinejad M, Kiger RD. A histologic evaluation of dental pulp tissue of a patient with periodontal disease. Oral Surg Oral Med Oral Pathol 1985;59:198–200.

54. Feiglin B. Pain and fistulas can cross the midline. J Endod 1985;11:132–134.

55. Kaufman AY. An enigmatic sinus tract origin. Endod Dent Traumatol 1989;5:159–161.

56. Cwyk F, Saint-Pierre F, Tronstad L. Endodontic implications of orthodontic tooth movement [abstract]. J Dent Res 1984;63:286.

57. Heithersay GS. Clinical, radiologic and histopathologic features of invasive cervical resorption. Quintessence Int 1999;30:27–37.

58. Tronstad L. Root resorption—Etiology, terminology and clinical manifestations. Endod Dent Traumatol 1988;4(6):241–252.

59. Goldman HM, Schilder H. Regeneration of attachment apparatus lost due to disease of endodontic origin. J Periodontol 1988;59:609–610.

60. Cardoso AS, Mitchell DF. Progression of pulpitis to necrosis and periapical disease in deciduous and permanent teeth of monkeys. J Dent Res 1971;50:934–938.

61. Walton RE, Pashley DH, Dowden WE. Pulp pathosis. In: Ingle JI (ed). Endodontics, ed 3. Philadelphia: Lea & Febiger, 1985.

62. Gorni F, Lamorgese V, Malentacca A. I riassorbimenti radicolari, I: Eziopatogenesi, diagnosi e manifestazioni cliniche. G Ital Endod 1991;5(2):36–42.

63. Marion CL. A clinical and histological investigation of the effects of periodontal curetage on the pulp with special emphasis on accessory canals [thesis]. Boston: Boston University, 1979.

64. Bergenholtz G, Lindhe J. Effect of experimentally induced marginal periodontitis and periodontal scaling on the dental pulp. J Clin Periodontol 1978;5:59–73.

65. Langeland K, Rodrigues H, Dowden W. Periodontal disease, bacteria, and pulpal histopathology. Oral Surg Oral Med Oral Pathol 1974;37:257–270.

66. Czarnecki RT. A histologic evaluation of the human pulp in teeth with varying degrees of periodontal disease [thesis]. Boston: Boston University, 1971.

67. Mascarello C, Marini R. La polpa dentaria nella malattia parodontale: Aspetti isto-patologici. L'Io & Ram 1990;9:8.

68. Hiatt WH. Periodontically and endontically involved teeth. In: Grossman LI (ed). Transactions of the Third International Conference on Endodontics. Philadelphia: University of Pennsylvania, 1963:201.

69. Waerhaug J. Healing of dento-epithelial function following subgingival plaque control, I: As observed in human biopsy material. J Periodontol 1978;49:1–8.

70. Waerhaug J. Healing of dento-epithelial function following subgingival plaque control, II: As observed on extracted teeth. J Periodontol 1978;49:119–134.

71. Rabbani GM, Ash MM, Caffesse RG. The effectiveness of subgingival scaling and root planing in calculus removal. J Periodontol 1981;52:119–123.

72. Carnevale GF, Pontoriero R, Di Febo GF. Long-term effects of root-resective therapy in furcation-involved molars. A 10-year longitudinal study. J Clin Periodontol 1998;25:209–214.

73. Tonetti M, Cortellini P, Suvan J et al. Generalizability of the added benefits of guided tissue regeneration in the treatment of deep intrabony defects. Evaluation in a multi-center randomized controlled clinical trial. J Periodontol 1998;69:1183–1192.

74. Milano F, Melsen B. Guided tissue regeneration using bioresorbable membranes: What is the limit in the treatment of combined periapical and marginal lesions? Int J Periodontics Restorative Dent 1997;17:416–425.

75. Nordernram A, Svärdström G. Results of apicoectomy. Swed Dent J 1970;63:593–604.

76. Beer R, Bauman MA, Kim S. Endodonzia. Milano: Masson, 1997.

77. Villa R, Rangert B. Early loading of interforaminal implants immediately installed after extraction of teeth presenting endodontic and periodontal lesions. Clin Implant Dent Relat Res 2005;7(suppl 1):S28–35.

78. Gelb DA. Immediate implant surgery: Three-year retrospective evaluation of 50 consecutive cases. Int J Oral Maxillofac Implants 1993;8:388–399.

79. Becker W, Becker BE, Polizzi G, Bergstrom C. Autogenous bone grafting of bone defects adjacent to implants placed into immediate extraction sockets in patients: A prospective study. Int J Oral Maxillofac Implants 1994;9:389–396.

80. Cornellini R, Barone A, Covani U, Wilson TG Jr. Implianti post estrattivi immediati: revisione della letteratura. Il Dentista Moderno 2006;8:42–47.

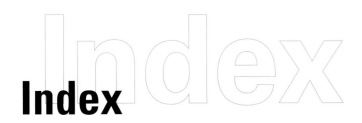

Index